AF886468

THE MEDICAL DEEP STATE

THE MEDICAL DEEP STATE

The Hidden System of Power That Is Hijacking Medicine and How Physicians Can Reclaim Control of Their Career and Calling

Curtis G. Graham, MD

Best Seller Publishing

Published by Best Seller Publishing®, St. Augustine, FL
Best Seller Publishing® is a registered trademark.
Printed in the United States of America.

ISBN: __________

For more information, please write:
Best Seller Publishing®
1775 US-1 #1070
St. Augustine, FL 32084
or call 1 (626) 765-9750

Visit us online at: www.BestSellerPublishing.org

ACKNOWLEDGMENTS

This book grew out of a long season of reckoning. What began as a personal effort to understand the decline in American healthcare has become something larger, an urgent call for physicians to ré-engage in shaping the system that affects both their lives and their patients' lives. I am grateful to those who helped me find the clarity and courage to write it.

My deepest thanks go to Bob Harpole, whose steady guidance shaped these pages into a form that invites readers into the complex and often hidden forces affecting modern medical practice. You stepped into a storm without warning and brought insight, patience, and an unwavering commitment to help tell this story.

I am also grateful for the friendship and sharp legal mind of Dirk Ravenholt, Attorney at Law. His thoughtful explanations of legal processes, courtroom realities, and principles of fairness gave me a clearer understanding of how physicians move within the boundaries of the law and sometimes cross them without intent. His counsel helped me frame these issues with more balance and common sense.

Finally, I want to acknowledge the growing body of writing that examines the crisis in healthcare and medical education. These contributions provided context, challenge, and confirmation as I traced the roots of the problems confronting our profession today.

To each person who contributed in ways large and small, thank you. Your support made this book possible.

Dedication

This book is dedicated to independent practicing physicians. I know the struggles you face because I have lived through them myself. I wrote these pages to share what I have learned in the hope that they offer clarity for the future, renewed reasons to stay in the profession, and fresh satisfaction in the value you bring to your patients. My wish is that you also find practical ways to guard against the forces that have driven so many physicians out of medicine.

Disclaimer

This book is based on the author's personal and professional experiences, opinions, and research. It is intended for informational and educational purposes only and should not be considered medical, legal, financial, or professional advice.

Readers, including physicians, should consult qualified professionals and business advisors before making decisions related to medical careers, finances, medical practice, licensing, or any form of healthcare delivery.

References to individuals or institutions, past or present, are drawn from real events but may have been altered to protect privacy. Every effort has been made to ensure the accuracy and appropriate dating of the information provided. The events, facts, and viewpoints described reflect the author's own experiences, research, and honest recollections. The views expressed are solely those of the author and do not represent the views of any organization with which the author is or has been affiliated.

TABLE OF CONTENTS

Preface: A Letter I Never Thought I'd Write 1

Introduction: A Profession at the Edge 5

PART 1: Diagnosis: A Profession in Crisis 7

Chapter 1: Why American Medicine Is Crumbling and Why It Matters Now 9

Chapter 2: The Education Gap What We Never Learned 13

Chapter 3: The Medical Deep State 21

Chapter 4: What Burnout Really Is and Why Physicians Hate That Word 33

Chapter 5: The Invisible Curriculum 37

Chapter 6: The Corporate Takeover of the Physician-Patient Relationship 41

Chapter 7: The Productivity Trap 49

PART 2: The Human Cost 53

Chapter 8: The Unseen Stakeholders 55

Chapter 9: The Training That Teaches Silence 57

Chapter 10: When Physicians Have No Voice 59

Chapter 11: When the System Profits from Silence....67

Chapter 12: The Consequences of Being Conditioned to Endure....71

Chapter 13: The Disillusionment of a Calling....75

Chapter 14: When There Are No Physicians Left....79

PART 3: Stakeholder Conversations....83

Chapter 15: To Hospital and Health System Leaders: Partner with Physicians, or Lose Them....85

Chapter 16: To Policymakers and Regulators: Regulate with, Not Over, Physicians....89

Chapter 17: To Medical Educators: Teach More Than Science....93

Chapter 18: To Medical Students and Residents: Stay Human, Stay Awake....97

Chapter 19: To Insurance Companies....101

Chapter 20: To Journalists and Media: Tell the Whole Story....105

Chapter 21: To Employers, Recruiters, and Contract Negotiators: Stop Exploiting the Naive....107

Chapter 22: To Private Practice Physicians: Your Autonomy Still Matters....109

Chapter 23: To Technology Leaders: Build with, Not Around, Physicians....115

Chapter 24: We Do What We Can and Hope for the Best....119

PART 4: Rebuilding Medicine from the Inside Out....123

Chapter 25: Solution: Eliminate Policy Structures That Harm....125

Chapter 26: Solution: Enforce Ethical Standards in Health Management 127

Chapter 27: Solution: Physician-Centered Technology 131

Chapter 28: Solution: A National Campaign for Physician Respect 133

Chapter 29: Solution: Compensation Models That Align with Purpose 135

Chapter 30: Solution: Restore Clinical Autonomy 139

Chapter 31: Solution: Business Literacy in Medical Training 143

Conclusion: We Still Have Time 147

Epilogue: What Nearly Broke Me: And What I Found on the Other Side 149

About the Author 153

PREFACE

A Letter I Never Thought I'd Write

Even now, it's hard to talk about what happened.

I was at the height of my career, leading a thriving OB/GYN practice, pioneering new procedures, and serving a community I cared deeply about. On the surface, I appeared to be successful. But beneath it, something was unraveling, not just for me but also for thousands of private practice physicians like me.

This unraveling isn't just about burnout. It's a preventable systemic failure. One that continues to hollow out our profession from the inside.

I lost my practice. And for a long time, I believed it was my fault. I thought I'd missed something. I reasoned that I wasn't strong enough. I figured that I'd failed.

But eventually, I began to see the truth: I was never given the tools to succeed. Like so many others, I was trained in medicine but sent into business.

And no one told me that those were two different things.

No medical school in this country teaches business, not in any meaningful, applied way. They'll say there's no time. The medical curriculum is already overloaded. But that's not the whole story.

Because what we're really being taught—through omission—is that we don't need that knowledge. That it's somehow beneath us. That if we're just good enough at medicine, everything else will work itself out.

It won't.

Running a private medical practice *is* running a business. You can't separate the two. And when physicians are sent out without that understanding, without support, and without the language even to know what questions to ask, we lose them. Quietly. Rapidly. Permanently.

In my own practice, I tried to figure it out on my own. I asked around. I gathered secondhand advice from other physicians. I pieced things together slowly by building an infertility program, investing in surgical training, and becoming the first in my state to perform advanced laparoscopic procedures. I even brought ultrasound technology into my office before anyone else in the region.

But none of that innovation could protect me from what I didn't know: billing systems, payer contracts, overhead calculations, legal traps buried in employment clauses, and the importance of cash flow. I was operating in the dark—and I didn't even know it.

Looking back, I see how easily it could have been different. If someone had pulled me aside and said, "*This is how the system actually works. These are the tools you need to navigate it. Here's how you protect your practice, your livelihood, your life.*" But no one did.

And now, I know I'm not alone. I've met countless physicians with the same story: skilled, compassionate, and driven—but unequipped. Many of them never recover. Some leave the profession entirely. Some lose their homes, their families, and their health. A few don't survive at all.

This is not a personal failure. It is a structural one.

And it has persisted, decade after decade, because of an outdated belief that physicians don't need business education. That our value lies solely in our clinical skill. That we can be good at one thing and ignore the rest.

That belief is destroying us.

We need a new model. One that recognizes physicians as both healers and professionals operating in a complex, high-stakes economy. One that teaches us how to read a contract, negotiate a fair salary, evaluate a practice model, and plan for financial sustainability. One that gives us power, not just knowledge.

I've waited years to say this publicly. Not because I was afraid, but because I didn't think it would matter. But I'm writing it now because I know that for some physician out there, who are reading this while barely holding it together, it *will* matter.

This letter is for you.

You're not failing. You're not broken. You're not alone.

And it's time we stop pretending that your collapse is a mystery. It's not. It's the predictable result of a system that sends brilliant, dedicated people into a career without providing them the tools to succeed.

Let's change that *together.*

INTRODUCTION

A Profession at the Edge

This book began with a question I could not stop asking: *Why are so many good physicians walking away?*

I have asked it in exam rooms, at dinner tables, on long drives home after another shift that ran too long. I have asked it to colleagues with tears in their eyes, to students full of doubt, and to myself in the quiet spaces where no one is listening.

The answers vary in detail but not in direction. The system has made it harder to care. Not harder to be smart. Not harder to be efficient. Harder to *care.* And that is what breaks physicians.

Because medicine is not just a job, it is a covenant. A trust between patient and healer. A moral calling carried out in the most intimate and uncertain moments of human life. When that calling is reduced to metrics, when policies undermine trust, and when human connection is interrupted by screens, something essential begins to erode.

We were not trained to endure that erosion. We were trained to fight it. But most of us were never taught how.

We were not taught how to negotiate our contracts. We were not taught how to lead teams, build practices, or navigate corporate strategy. We were not taught how to recognize moral injury, how to advocate without fear of punishment, or how to thrive in systems that prioritize output over wisdom.

And so, we burn out. We fall silent. We retreat into compliance or resignation. Or we leave.

This book is for those who have stayed, and for those who might still return. It is for the medical student beginning to wonder if the dream was naive. It is for the resident who no longer feels safe speaking up. It is for the mid-career physician who feels trapped between what they believe and what they are allowed to do. It is for the leader who wants to improve but doesn't know where to start.

And it is for the people outside the profession who shape the conditions in which medicine happens. Lawmakers. Executives. Educators. Journalists. Patients. Every one of them plays a role in this story.

This is not a memoir. It is not an academic treatise. It is a call to remember what medicine is supposed to be, as well as a map of what must change for us to reclaim it.

The chapters ahead address different audiences, propose various solutions, and highlight distinct problems. But they are united by one conviction: We cannot save the profession without listening to those who live it. Not through surveys. Not through committees. But rather, through real engagement, real partnership, and real courage.

If you are looking for easy answers, you will not find them here. But if you are looking for truth told plainly, if you are willing to wrestle with complexity, if you still believe that medicine can be what it was meant to be, then you are not alone.

The profession is not lost. But it is at the edge.

And it is time to decide which way we will go.

Part 1

Diagnosis: A Profession in Crisis

CHAPTER 1

Why American Medicine Is Crumbling and Why It Matters Now

If future physicians were introduced to economic reality, the medical profession might cease to be part of the cost problem and become part of the solution.

—John G. Freymann, MD,
National Fund for Medical Education

In the past, the phrase "American physician" conjured an image of competence, respect, and resilience: a profession built on sacrifice, excellence, and trust. But something foundational is cracking. A growing number of physicians, once drawn to medicine by a sense of calling, are quietly walking away. Others stay but feel trapped, exhausted, overregulated, and disillusioned. We are living through a slow, barely acknowledged collapse of one of the most vital professions in our country.

It is tempting to think this is a temporary setback, a cyclical low point that will reverse itself with time. But the data, as well as the lived experiences of thousands of physicians, tell a different story. Fewer young people are applying to medical school, especially men. Those who do make it through the gauntlet of training often enter a career that quickly feels unsustainable. Burnout is no longer the exception. It is the expectation.

Everywhere you look, the profession is fraying. Family practices are disappearing from entire states. Suicide rates among physicians are climbing. Staffing shortages aren't so much a looming threat as they are a present crisis. Yet this unraveling rarely makes headlines. It shows up in the quiet resignation of a solo practice shuttered after decades, in a physician sobbing in the supply closet, or in a boardroom where no one hears the clinician's voice.

> *The physician is expected to meet the grim monster, break the jaws of death, and pluck the spoil out of his teeth.*
>
> —R. V. Pierce, MD, President, World's Dispensary Medical Association, Buffalo, NY (1895)

The reasons for this collapse are layered and complex. But one truth surfaces again and again: We have trained physicians to diagnose disease, but not to navigate the system in which they must practice. We have taught them how to save lives, but not how to sustain their own.

Medical education in America prizes scientific rigor, clinical skill, and intellectual stamina. These qualities remain essential, but no longer are they enough. Physicians today are expected not only to provide care but also to manage businesses, decipher insurance contracts, comply with an ever-expanding maze of regulations, meet productivity quotas, and absorb the weight of a broken infrastructure. Yet none of these responsibilities are meaningfully addressed in their training.

We have created an education system that equips physicians to treat illness but not to survive the profession. In this knowledge vacuum, a troubling pattern has emerged: The more clinically skilled a physician is, the more vulnerable they may be in a system that treats them like interchangeable labor rather than autonomous professionals.

I know this pattern firsthand.

Early in my career, I built a thriving OB/GYN practice. I stayed up-to-date on the science. I loved my patients. I did the work with heart and integrity. I believed that clinical excellence would protect me. That belief collapsed the day I walked into a licensing board meeting, expecting a routine approval for a license in a new state. Instead, I was blindsided by a physician board member (likely not even from my specialty), who used an old case to deliver a scathing ten-minute critique. I had honored a patient's decision to avoid a C-section. The baby had been born healthy. No complaints were ever filed.

But I wasn't allowed to respond. There was no process for context, no legal counsel, no defense. The board denied my license on the spot. The damage didn't stop there. Other states took notice. Malpractice insurers backed away. The career I had spent decades building unraveled.

It wasn't a medical failure that ended my practice. It was a lack of preparation for how the system actually works: the politics, the perception, the power structures that govern medicine outside the exam room. I had no tools to navigate any of it.

What I had encountered was not just a confusing bureaucracy or a one-off injustice. It was part of something much larger and more insidious. It was part of a coordinated, profit-driven web of interests that shape the rules of the game. Throughout this book, I refer to it as the Medical Deep State. It is not a shadowy conspiracy, but rather a deeply entrenched network of predators, including insurance companies, corporate hospital systems, regulatory boards, data vendors, and silent stakeholders who benefit from physician disempowerment. Their presence is not always visible, but their influence shows up in every absurd reimbursement rule, every burned-out colleague, and every barrier that keeps doctors from doing what they were trained to do: care for patients.

And that is the deeper crisis. Not that the system is flawed (although it is), but we continue to send physicians into that system unequipped, unsupported, and unaware of the dangers they may face. The system doesn't just punish clinical mistakes. It punishes administrative missteps, bureaucratic naivety, and ethical decisions that challenge corporate convenience.

Some critics have framed this crisis as a generational problem. They say younger physicians are too sensitive, too entitled, unwilling to work hard. But that's a distraction. The profession is not struggling because physicians are weaker. It is struggling because the environment around them has become increasingly hostile to the kind of medicine that drew them to the field in the first place.

At the heart of this problem is one avoidable failure: the absence of business, legal, and leadership education in medical training. It's as if we trained pilots to fly but never taught them to read the fuel gauge or manage an emergency landing. We cling to the noble idea that medicine is a calling, not a business. But that distinction, while romantic, is dangerous. The refusal to teach physicians how to lead, how to negotiate, how to read a contract, how to manage risk—that refusal is costing us dearly.

This book is not a lament. It is a call to action and a blueprint for change.

We do not need another pep talk. We need a reckoning. A new model for educating and supporting physicians—one that empowers them not just to practice medicine, but to survive and lead within it.

Because behind every struggling physician is a suffering patient. Behind every closed practice is a community with less access to care. And behind every silent resignation is a story that could have ended differently, if only we had dared to teach our physicians not just how to heal others, but how to protect themselves.

Let's do better. Not someday. Now.

CHAPTER 2

The Education Gap What We Never Learned

If a physician invested one hour every day doing nothing but thinking, brainstorming, creating new and better ways to be of greater and more valued service to his medical patients, money problems would melt away.

—Earl Nightingale

By every traditional measure, medical education in the United States is a triumph. It is rigorous, intellectually demanding, and grounded in science. It prepares students to recognize rare diseases, interpret complex lab results, and perform intricate procedures. It produces professionals who can think clearly in a crisis, endure long hours, and shoulder immense responsibility.

And yet, for all its brilliance, it fails in one crucial way.

Medical education trains physicians to practice medicine, but not to live inside the profession.

From the first day of anatomy lab to the last day of residency, students are taught that medicine is a calling. They are taught to persevere, to master knowledge, and to put patients first. They are trained to deliver care in crisis settings, make life-altering decisions under pressure, and memorize more material than many thought possible. But almost nothing in that journey prepares them for what happens after the training ends.

They are not taught how to read a contract. They are not taught how to choose between employment models or what to look for in a partnership agreement. They are not taught how to manage a budget, lead a team, bill ethically, or protect themselves from burnout. And they are certainly not taught how to navigate the political, legal, and economic forces that now shape almost every aspect of clinical life.

> *The cause of man's problem is lack of knowledge. It does not stem from a shortage of information, but from rejections of information.*
>
> —Hosea 4:6 (paraphrase)

These gaps in training are not accidental. They serve what I call the Medical Deep State, which is a network of power that depends on physicians being uninformed. The less we know about contracts, laws, billing, or systems management, the easier we are to control. From the first day of training, the profession is shaped to fit into that machine without ever being told it exists.

The result? Medical students learn to save lives, but not how to sustain their own.

Why Physicians Didn't See It Coming

Over the past century of modern medical practice, physicians have experienced a steady expansion of responsibility, regulation, documentation, and financial pressure. What is notable is not simply the growth of these demands, but the absence of any sustained institutional effort to reduce them. The reduction of physician workload, administrative burden, or economic vulnerability has never been treated as a central objective of modern healthcare. Instead, physicians have been expected to adapt to increasing complexity as a normal condition of practice.

The consequences of this approach have accumulated gradually. Independent medical practices have become more difficult to sustain, professional dissatisfaction has increased, and physician burnout and attrition are now widely regarded as unavoidable features of modern medicine rather than as indicators of systemic failure. Yet this deterioration did not emerge suddenly. The warning signs were present long before physicians reached exhaustion or disengagement.

One factor has received far less attention than it warrants: the absence of meaningful business education in medical training. For generations, physicians have entered practice exceptionally well prepared to deliver medical care, but largely unprepared to operate within the financial and organizational realities that shape modern healthcare. Most begin their careers with little understanding of pricing structures, contractual leverage, cost controls, or long-term practice sustainability. This gap is neither incidental nor rare; it has been a persistent feature of medical education.

As a result, early indicators of trouble are often misunderstood. Patient volumes plateau or decline. Practice income stagnates despite longer hours and increasing administrative demands. Expenses continue to rise. The typical response is to work harder, see more patients, or accept additional obligations in the belief that increased effort will restore stability. In many cases, it does not. The underlying dynamics remain unchanged, and the pressure intensifies.

Over time, physicians may recognize that something is no longer working, but they lack the framework needed to identify the source of the problem. Clinical skill, dedication, and ethical commitment do not automatically translate into economic security or professional autonomy. The realization that excellence alone is insufficient can be deeply unsettling and often marks a turning point in a physician's relationship with their work.

Burnout commonly follows, but it is important to understand it correctly. Burnout is not the initiating cause of professional collapse; it is the end stage. It reflects prolonged exposure to financial and structural pressures that physicians were never trained to manage or even fully recognize.

What deserves careful attention is how long this pattern has persisted. Medical schools, professional organizations, and healthcare leadership have been aware of rising physician stress and attrition for decades. Yet the foundational vulnerability—lack of business literacy—has remained largely unaddressed. Physicians have instead been encouraged to cultivate resilience or adjust expectations, responses that may offer temporary relief but do not alter the conditions producing the strain.

The erosion of independent medical practice carries consequences beyond individual careers. It affects patient access, continuity of care, and the long-term stability of the healthcare system itself. Until physicians are equipped to understand and navigate the non-clinical forces shaping their practices, they will remain exposed to pressures that are difficult to see, difficult to measure, and difficult to resist.

The consequences of that omission are neither abstract nor rare. Some manage to figure it out through mentors or trial and error. Others don't. They walk into practice naive about the business of medicine, unprepared for the bureaucracy, and unaware that a single misunderstanding or a vindictive reviewer can jeopardize their license and reputation. It is not just an education gap. It is a setup.

Physicians are not failing because they lack intelligence or commitment. They are failing because no one ever showed them how the system actually works. Here is how that gap looks in practice:

- Signing payer, hospital, and private equity contracts that hide unfair terms.
- Losing 10 to 25 percent of revenue because of coding errors or denial blind spots.

- Having no offense or defense strategy for prior authorization or appeals.
- Allowing others to define value-based care rules and keep the surplus.

These are not small oversights. They are structural blind spots that weaken physicians at the exact points where they need strength. A curriculum that closes these gaps is not optional. It is survival. Here is what a minimum business curriculum could look like if we had the courage to build it:

1. **Health finance and accounting.** Learn how the revenue cycle works, how to model payer mix, and how to track cash flow.
2. **Contracting and negotiation.** Read payer agreements, employment contracts, and private equity deals with clarity.
3. **Coding, risk, and quality.** Master E/M coding, risk adjustment, and audit defense.
4. **Regulatory and legal.** Understand Stark, Anti-Kickback, HIPAA, and state corporate practice laws.
5. **Practice operations.** Build staffing models, manage schedules, and control supply costs.
6. **Prior authorization and utilization.** Use templated necessity language and appeal ladders.
7. **Data and analytics.** Create dashboards, analyze denial trends, and scorecard payers.
8. **Leadership and HR.** Hire well, design incentives, and track burnout prevention as a KPI.
9. **Marketing and patient access.** Build referral networks and protect access.
10. **Entrepreneurship and private equity literacy.** Read MSO structures and equity terms.
11. **Capstone.** Build a pro forma, negotiate a contract amendment, and defend a mock audit.

If physicians graduate without these skills, they enter the profession already at a disadvantage. That is not education. That is abandonment.

I remember what it felt like to emerge from training with the confidence of someone who had done the hard work. I'd delivered babies, managed emergencies, and studied relentlessly. I'd done everything asked of me. I built a practice, earned respect, and built trust with my patients. But I had never been taught the rules behind the rules.

Years later, when a licensing board denied me the right to practice in another state based on a mischaracterized case, I realized just how exposed I was. I had no legal counsel. No playbook. No understanding of how easily the system could turn on me, not because of poor medicine, but because of politics and perception. What I needed was not another CME on managing preeclampsia. What I needed was a course on survival.

My story is not unique. It is being repeated across the country every day, in small and large ways. New physicians step into the real world and find themselves overwhelmed, not by the medicine but everything else. They don't know what the codes on their paycheck mean. They don't know how to challenge a wrongful denial of payment. They don't know how to protect themselves from legal exposure. And because they don't know what they don't know, they often don't realize the danger until it's too late.

We have trained physicians to master uncertainty in the clinical realm, but not in the business realm. And the result is a generation of MDs who are brilliant in the exam room but vulnerable in the boardroom.

There are bright spots. A few schools have begun offering elective courses in leadership or practice management. A few residencies bring in guest speakers to discuss contracts or burnout. But these efforts are inconsistent, underfunded, and often optional. And even when they exist, they are rarely integrated into the core curriculum.

That must change.

We need to teach business literacy as rigorously as we teach pathophysiology. We need to treat practice management, negotiation, personal finance, and systems navigation as essential competencies. We need to prepare physicians not only to enter the profession but also to thrive in it.

The gap is not just educational. It is ethical. If we continue to graduate physicians without the tools to protect themselves, we are complicit in their vulnerability. If we expect them to survive a system we never taught them to understand, we are setting them up to fail.

This chapter is a call for reform, not to dilute the clinical rigor of medical training but to expand its definition of what it means to be truly prepared. The best physicians are not only skilled in diagnosis. They are equipped to lead, to advocate, to sustain themselves in the face of pressure.

Until we treat business education as essential to physician development, we will continue to lose some of our best minds to a system they were never taught to survive.

CHAPTER 3

The Medical Deep State

When physicians enter practice without the tools to understand the business environment surrounding them, financial pressure rarely announces itself as a single disruptive event. Instead, it accumulates gradually through ordinary interactions that appear legitimate, contractual, and routine. Over time, these interactions extract income, time, and autonomy from independent medical practices in ways that are difficult to recognize without deliberate scrutiny.

This erosion does not require coordination or malicious intent. It is driven by incentives. Every vendor, supplier, service company, and corporate entity in healthcare is structured to maximize its own revenue and growth. Independent physician practices, lacking business literacy and internal oversight, are especially vulnerable to these pressures. Each actor operates independently, yet the cumulative effect is substantial and sustained.

Most physicians do not routinely audit the non-clinical side of their practices. Product pricing is rarely verified against invoices. Service fees are accepted without challenge. Billing discrepancies go unnoticed. Contracts are renewed automatically. Few practices track incremental overcharges or assess whether costs align with value received. Individually, these losses may seem negligible. Collectively, they erode a practice's financial stability over time.

Medical service companies understand this dynamic. They know physicians are focused on patient care, not vendor oversight. Pricing structures, bundled services, and periodic fee adjustments are often designed to increase margins quietly and incrementally. In the absence of internal review or independent comparison, these practices persist unchecked. What appears to be administrative noise becomes a consistent drain on revenue.

Pharmaceutical companies provide one clear illustration of how legitimate business strategies can reshape physician behavior without explicit agreement or compensation. When direct-to-consumer advertising expanded in the late twentieth century, it demonstrated the financial power of influencing public demand. Providing free product samples to physician offices extended that strategy. Physicians, acting in good faith, distributed samples without recognizing that they were also performing unpaid marketing labor.

When a physician hands a patient a sample medication, that action carries implicit endorsement. Patients often continue the same product once the sample is finished, reinforcing brand loyalty established at no cost to the manufacturer. The physician invests time, storage space, and clinical authority, yet receives no compensation while assuming additional administrative burden. Over time, these small, uncompensated activities add to the cumulative strain on independent practices.

Pharmaceuticals are not unique in this regard. They are illustrative. Similar dynamics exist across vendor contracts, billing services, data platforms, equipment suppliers, and administrative intermediaries. The common feature is asymmetry: One party designs the terms, while the other absorbs the complexity.

None of these mechanisms are hidden. They are embedded within standard business relationships and accepted industry norms. Their effectiveness depends not on secrecy, but on normalization. Without training in negotiation, cost analysis, and contract management, physicians are rarely positioned to question or counter these arrangements. What appears to be partnership often functions as unequal exchange.

This is the operational reality of what I refer to as the Medical Deep State. It is not a shadow organization or centralized authority. It is a network of financial and administrative structures whose incentives align around physician disengagement from the business side of medicine. Its power lies in accumulation—in advantages gained incrementally, contract by contract, invoice by invoice, until imbalance becomes the default condition.

Understanding these mechanisms changes what is possible. Without that understanding, physicians may work longer hours, see more patients, and sacrifice more of themselves without improving the sustainability of their practices. With it, they gain the capacity to recognize extraction, question assumptions, and begin restoring balance to their professional lives.

What We Mean by the Medical Deep State

What you have just seen is not accidental. It reflects a system I have already mentioned more than once—the Medical Deep State. By that, I do not mean a shadowy conspiracy or a secret cabal pulling strings in the dark. Rather, I mean the web of entrenched powers and interests that now dominate American medicine. This is what shapes the conditions in which physicians practice, often invisibly, yet with enormous impact on our daily work and on the choices we are allowed to make.

If we are going to understand why physicians are leaving the profession in such alarming numbers, we cannot stop with surface explanations like burnout or exhaustion. Those are real, but they are symptoms. The deeper truth is that medicine has been captured by outside forces that benefit when physicians are kept in a position of dependence. The result is a profession in which doctors are trained to heal but systematically stripped of the ability to control their own futures.

This chapter is an attempt to name and describe that system. I want to explain what the Medical Deep State is, what it is not, where it came from, and how it continues to shape the profession today. You will see how historical decisions, regulatory frameworks, and corporate strategies have combined to build an environment in which physicians feel trapped and disempowered.

Only by examining this hidden architecture can we make sense of why the profession has eroded so dramatically in such a short span of time. And only by naming it clearly can we begin to imagine a path forward that restores physicians to their rightful place in the center of American healthcare.

How It Took Hold

The Medical Deep State did not spring up overnight. It was built piece by piece, policy by policy, over the course of more than a century. Each change was presented as progress, and in some ways it was, but the cumulative effect was to draw physicians further away from independence and deeper into dependence on outside powers.

A turning point came with the Flexner Report in 1910. It reformed standardized medical education and raised scientific rigor, which undoubtedly improved patient care. But in narrowing the curriculum to focus almost exclusively on the sciences, it stripped away any recognition that medicine also functions within a business and legal environment. From that moment on, physicians were trained to practice medicine as if the practice itself existed in isolation, untouched by economics or policy. The seeds of vulnerability were planted.

Decades later, the introduction of Medicare and Medicaid transformed the way medicine was paid for. These programs opened access to care for millions of Americans, but they also made government the dominant payer and pulled physicians into a web of regulations and reimbursement rules. The relationship between doctor and patient was no longer only about clinical judgment, but now required constant negotiation with bureaucratic systems that cared as much about paperwork as about outcomes.

The HMO Act of 1973 deepened this shift. Managed care placed insurers at the center of decision-making and stripped physicians of authority over treatment plans. What began as an effort to control costs quickly became a mechanism of control over physicians themselves. Doctors found their clinical choices filtered through utilization reviews and prior authorizations, tools that grew in power with every passing decade.

Regulation and compliance continued to expand. HIPAA, while vital for privacy, imposed enormous administrative costs that fell hardest on small private practices. Then the Affordable Care Act accelerated hospital consolidation, swallowing up independent practices and forcing many physicians into employment contracts that tied their futures to the interests of health systems rather than patients.

None of these reforms were designed to destroy physician independence outright. Yet when placed together, they created exactly that effect. Each law and regulation shifted a little more control away from the exam room and toward outside entities. By the time many physicians realized what had happened, the environment of medicine had been rewritten around them. What was once a profession rooted in trust and autonomy had become a system in which doctors were measured, managed, and often silenced by powers they could not see but felt at every turn.

How It Operates Today

The result of those historical shifts is the system physicians live inside right now. It is not simply the long hours or the emotional toll of caring for patients that drives so many from the profession. It is the relentless pressure of outside forces dictating how medicine is practiced. Physicians wake up every day to an obstacle course designed by industries that depend on their labor while steadily eroding their autonomy.

Insurance companies stand at the center of this environment. They determine which treatments will be approved, what will be reimbursed, and how much time and money physicians must spend appealing denials that have little to do with clinical judgment. Each prior authorization, each rejection of a claim, each delay in payment shifts the balance of power away from the physician and toward a corporation that profits by saying no.

Hospitals and health systems have become another source of control. Through consolidation, they have transformed physicians from independent professionals into employees bound by restrictive contracts. Decisions about staffing, scheduling, and referral patterns are often made by administrators whose first priority is revenue rather than patient care. Physicians who once built practices that reflected their values now find themselves answering to business executives who measure them by volume and compliance rather than wisdom and compassion.

The pharmaceutical and device industries add another layer. Their influence reaches into prescribing habits, practice guidelines, and even the education of physicians. What is presented as innovation or support often doubles as marketing. Physicians become both the customer and the product, caught in a cycle in which their recommendations serve corporate strategies as much as patient needs.

Overlaying all of this is a vast regulatory apparatus. Each year brings new reporting requirements, new compliance rules, and new penalties for falling short. What is promised as accountability often becomes a trap, shifting costs and risks onto physicians who are already stretched to their limits. The culture of medicine, once rooted in trust, is steadily replaced by a culture of surveillance and documentation.

This is how the Medical Deep State operates in the present. It does not announce itself or claim a single face. It functions through policies, contracts, and incentives that together drain physicians of control over their own profession. *Burnout* may be the word that captures the symptoms, but the cause is systemic exploitation.

Physicians are not exhausted because they lack resilience. They are exhausted because they are asked to serve a machine that thrives on their compliance and profits from their silence.

Why Physicians Were Left Defenseless

If the Medical Deep State has been able to grow so powerful, it is not only because of corporate strength or regulatory complexity. It is also because physicians were never given the tools to resist it. From the very beginning of training, we were prepared to master medicine but not the world in which medicine must function.

Medical school demanded long hours, relentless study, and the ability to endure stress that few professions can imagine. Residency trained us to respond in crisis, to make rapid decisions under pressure, and to put patients first, no matter the cost to ourselves. What it did not teach us, however, was how to read a contract, how to manage a budget, how to protect ourselves legally, or how to negotiate with institutions that do not share our priorities.

This gap was not accidental. By stripping business education from the curriculum, the system created a workforce of highly skilled professionals who remained economically and legally naive. That naivety made us easy to control. It meant that when an insurer denied payment or a hospital demanded compliance, we often had no strategy and no vocabulary to resist.

I remember what it felt like when I stepped out of training with the confidence of someone who had done everything asked of him. I had studied, worked, sacrificed, and built a practice I believed in. But when I faced a licensing board that questioned my judgment, I realized I had no playbook for survival. I had never been taught how to defend myself against a system that could strip away my livelihood with a single vote. My ignorance was not unique. It was built into the way we train physicians in this country.

This is why so many of us were blindsided when the profession began to collapse around us. We had no way to understand the contracts we signed, the coding rules we were expected to follow, or the regulatory structures that governed our every move. The education gap became a weakness that the Deep State exploited with precision.

Physicians were not undone because they lacked intelligence or resilience. They were undone because they were sent into a complex and hostile environment without the training to navigate it. That failure of preparation has become one of the deepest betrayals of modern medicine.

What This Means for Patients and the Nation

The collapse of physician independence is not just a professional crisis. It reaches far beyond individual careers and touches the very foundation of healthcare in the United States. When physicians leave medicine or surrender their autonomy, the consequences fall directly on patients and communities.

Access to care is already fragile in many parts of the country. Rural areas that once relied on small physician-owned practices now struggle as those practices vanish. Patients who could once see the same doctor for years are forced into systems where continuity is broken and where they become numbers in a queue rather than people in a relationship. The loss of physician-led care has left entire communities without a trusted advocate in moments of deepest need.

The economic costs are just as damaging. Corporate systems that replace physician-owned practices rarely deliver care more efficiently. Instead, they layer administrative costs on top of clinical work, driving expenses higher while outcomes stagnate. Patients feel this in the form of rising premiums, higher deductibles, and more frequent denials of care. What was once a profession guided by judgment and compassion has become a business guided by spreadsheets, and the public pays the price.

Trust, too, is eroded. When physicians are treated as interchangeable providers under the authority of institutions, patients sense the loss of independence. They notice when doctors spend more time staring at screens than listening. They see when care is delayed by prior authorizations or restricted by formularies. The bond of trust.

that has always been the heart of medicine weakens, and without it, both physician and patient suffer.

This erosion of the profession is not just a matter of efficiency or convenience. It poses a risk to the health of the nation. Physician shortages are projected to grow in the coming decade, leaving millions without adequate access to care. Innovation slows when independent physicians, once free to experiment and pioneer, are folded into rigid corporate systems. In the long run, the disappearance of physician autonomy threatens not just individual health outcomes but the resilience of the entire healthcare system.

The crisis we face is not confined to burnout statistics or professional dissatisfaction. It is a matter of public well-being and national security. If physicians cannot survive in this environment, then neither can the patients who depend on them.

The Path Forward

If the Medical Deep State has hollowed out the profession, then the only way forward is to confront it directly. That will not happen through more slogans about wellness or resilience. It will not come from another task force that studies burnout while ignoring its causes. The path forward requires rebuilding the foundation of medicine so that physicians are no longer defenseless inside their own profession.

The first step is education. Business, finance, law, and leadership must become part of the medical curriculum, not as electives but as core competencies. Physicians should graduate with the ability to read a contract, understand a revenue cycle, lead a team, and protect themselves from exploitation. Without these skills, every new generation enters the profession unprepared for the world that waits for them.

The second step is independence. We must support models of practice that allow physicians to lead their own clinics and networks. Direct primary care, physician-owned groups, and community-based practices offer alternatives to corporate employment that preserve autonomy and restore patient trust. These models need protection and encouragement rather than the constant pressure of consolidation and buyout.

The third step is reform. Regulation must be simplified so that accountability strengthens care rather than suffocates it. Prior authorization should be stripped of its power to delay necessary treatment. Liability should be distributed fairly rather than concentrated on individual physicians. Transparency must become the rule, exposing how money and influence flow through insurers, hospitals, and pharmaceutical companies.

Finally, we must reclaim the cultural identity of physicians. We are not providers or interchangeable parts in a system. We are professionals with a calling, leaders in our communities, and stewards of public trust. Restoring that identity is not nostalgia. It is survival. Without it, the profession will continue to fracture until there is nothing left worth preserving.

The Deep State in medicine has grown powerful because it has operated quietly, feeding on physician vulnerability and public inattention. It can no longer remain unnamed. To confront it is not only to defend the dignity of physicians but also to safeguard the future of American healthcare. The path forward will not be easy, but it is necessary. Without bold action, the profession will continue to lose its best and brightest. With it, we have a chance to reclaim medicine for those who chose it not as a job, but as a life's work.

The Medical Deep State is not a theory. It is the reality that frames every decision a physician makes today. By naming it, tracing its rise, and exposing its impact, we can finally begin to see the true enemy of the profession. But naming it is only the beginning. In the chapters ahead, we will turn from diagnosis to prescription, from identifying the forces that have weakened medicine to exploring how we can equip physicians with the tools and strategies to reclaim their profession and restore the covenant between doctor and patient.

But before turning to solutions, we need to be clear about what kind of posture this moment demands of physicians themselves. Recognizing how independent medical practices are weakened is necessary, but recognition alone is not enough. Awareness without agency leads to frustration, cynicism, or disengagement. The goal is not simply to see the system more clearly, but to re-enter it with discernment, leverage, and intention.

Business literacy is often misunderstood as a departure from medicine's ethical core. In reality, it is an extension of it. A physician who cannot sustain a practice cannot sustain patient care. Financial instability compromises judgment, limits access, and accelerates burnout. Protecting the integrity of one's practice is not a distraction from patient care; it is a prerequisite for it.

Many physicians respond to pressure by working harder, sacrificing more time, and accepting additional obligations. This instinct is understandable, but it is often counterproductive. Increased effort within a structurally imbalanced system tends to amplify extraction rather than resolve it. Endurance, when it substitutes for insight, benefits those who profit from physician exhaustion.

Agency begins with understanding. When physicians learn how contracts are structured, how revenue is generated and lost, how incentives shape behavior, and how risk is transferred, their posture changes. They ask different questions. They recognize when compliance is optional rather than mandatory. They negotiate rather than absorb. They design systems instead of reacting to them.

This shift does not require abandoning medicine or rejecting institutions wholesale. It requires refusing the false choice between idealism and survival. Physicians can remain deeply committed to patient care while also insisting on fairness, transparency, and sustainability. Independence, in this sense, is not isolation. It is informed participation.

The Medical Deep State depends not on physician incompetence, but on physician disengagement from the business realities that govern their work. Re-engagement that is deliberate, informed, and strategic is the antidote. Education transforms confusion into clarity and resentment into resolve.

The future of medicine will not be secured by endurance alone. It will be shaped by physicians who understand the systems they work within and who choose to lead rather than simply survive them.

CHAPTER 4

What Burnout Really Is and Why Physicians Hate That Word

The word *burnout* is everywhere. In headlines. In HR training. In town halls hosted by hospital executives. It is the term we reach for when the people doing the most challenging work begin to crack under the weight of it. It has become the universal diagnosis for a workforce in distress.

But among physicians, the word often lands with a thud. Not because it is inaccurate, but because it is incomplete. It feels like a label slapped on a gaping wound. It describes the symptoms but obscures the cause.

Physician burnout is not just exhaustion. It is betrayal. It is the cumulative toll of practicing in a system that undermines your ability to do the work well and then blames you for feeling the strain.

When physicians speak privately, they rarely say, "I'm burned out." They say things like, "I can't keep doing this." Or "I dread going to work." Or "I feel like a cog in a machine that doesn't care what I think or how hard I try."

What they are describing is not a personal failure. It is a systemic malfunction. Calling it burnout without naming the conditions that cause it is like diagnosing smoke and ignoring the fire.

I remember that feeling vividly. After years of clinical excellence and patient dedication, I found myself staring at a licensing board that seemed more interested in optics than in truth. They had brought an accusation against me and had the outcome already decided. Although I had followed correct protocols in the delivery of a baby, years later I was accused of mishandling the case. I was summarily judged without even having a chance to effectively present my side of the story.

The rage I felt was not just about the injustice of the decision. It was about the realization that the system I had trusted to be fair and rational was anything but. I had played by the rules. And still, I was punished.

That experience was my first personal encounter with the Medical Deep State. It is not a shadowy cabal. It is the weight of boards, payers, regulators, attorneys, and political interests pressing on the exam room from the outside. They do not need to conspire in secret. Their influence is already woven into policy and paperwork, and that influence carries real power.

This is the force that allows physicians to be punished despite doing everything right. It is what turns honest clinical judgment into grounds for discipline. It is what transforms a moment of patient advocacy into a professional liability. The Medical Deep State does not need to be malicious to do harm. It simply needs to function as it was built, which is to protect the system, not the people in it.

That moment marked the beginning of a deeper unraveling—not just of my career trajectory but also of my belief that being a good physician was enough. I loved the work. But the system had made it impossible to love how the work was being treated.

This is the story behind much of what gets labeled *burnout.* It is not just about long hours or complex patients. Physicians expect those. What they do not expect—what they cannot tolerate indefinitely—

is being asked to uphold standards of care in systems that make good care harder and harder to deliver.

They do not burn out because they lack resilience. They burn out because they are forced to choose daily between what their patients need and what the system allows. They burn out because they are told they are autonomous professionals, only to be treated as replaceable workers. They burn out because they are trying to carry a moral weight that their institutions no longer seem willing to share.

But there's another layer too, one that lives beneath the surface of policy and structure. Burnout isn't simply about what the system does to physicians. It's also about what happens when the system never asks who the physician is in the first place.

After years of studying the rising mistreatment and burnout among physicians, I began to see a layer of the problem that most discussions overlook. Beneath the surface of policy failures, administrative overload, and economic pressures lies a more personal and often unspoken reality. Medical education and institutional leadership have rarely acknowledged, let alone explored, the role that a physician's individual traits and limitations play in how they endure the pressures of practice. It's as if we've designed a system that assumes all physicians are the same, or should be. But they're not.

Every physician carries a different threshold for stress, a unique way of adapting to challenge, and a set of emotional and psychological boundaries. Some can function for long stretches without sleep. Others struggle deeply with isolation or bureaucratic minutiae. Some are energized by the chaos of emergency care, while others thrive in quiet, methodical environments. Yet in all my years, I've never seen a structured effort to identify these personal distinctions during training, nor to use them as a guide when helping physicians choose a specialty or career path that truly fits them.

We test for knowledge. We train for skill. But we rarely assess the person behind the credentials. As a result, we send physicians into specialties or practice settings that might work against their natural temperament or endurance. I've known brilliant OB/GYNs who dreaded surgery. Interns who couldn't be roused during overnight calls. Internists who insisted on controlling every committee conversation, and others who withdrew completely when under pressure. These were not failures of intelligence or effort. They were mismatches between the person and the demands placed upon them.

If we could recognize our own weak points early—that is, if the system gave us the language and support to do so—we might be able to guide more physicians into roles that amplify their strengths instead of exposing their vulnerabilities. That would not only protect their well-being; it would also strengthen the entire profession. We lose too many good doctors not because they lack ability, but because we never asked whether they were in the right place to begin with.

And when physicians begin to feel the strain of that mismatch, the support they receive often misses the mark entirely. Wellness programs. Mindfulness apps. Time management workshops. These may be well-intentioned, but they often come across as dismissive. They suggest that the problem lies within the physician, rather than in the structure of the work itself.

Real solutions start with listening to physicians and asking what is depleting them, and then acting on their responses. By restoring their ability to influence how care is delivered. By protecting time for reflection, connection, and complexity, and honoring the fact that medicine is not a transaction. It is a relationship.

The word *burnout* may persist. It is short. It is catchy. It gets attention. But if we are serious about healing medicine, we must be serious about what the word obscures. And we must be willing to name the truth that every burned-out physician is trying to live through: that the system is not just taking their time. It is taking their trust.

And without trust, nothing in medicine works for long.

CHAPTER 5

The Invisible Curriculum

If you have a poor financial education, you will always work for the rich.

—Robert Kiyosaki, entrepreneur and investor

Every physician remembers the official curriculum of medical school: anatomy labs, pharmacology lectures, clinical rotations, and standardized patients. These are the building blocks of medical knowledge, the visible syllabus that shapes the first years of training.

But beneath that formal structure lies another education. It is less visible, less acknowledged, but no less powerful. It is the hidden curriculum—the set of implicit lessons and values that shape how future MDs learn to think, behave, and see themselves.

The hidden curriculum teaches you which specialties are respected and which are mocked. It teaches you how to stay awake for 36 hours without complaining. It teaches you to suppress your emotions, to see patients as cases, and to measure your worth by how much you can endure.

It teaches you, above all, that asking for help is a weakness. That struggling means you're not cut out for this. That vulnerability is dangerous.

This curriculum is not written down anywhere, but it is enforced with brutal consistency. It lives in the sarcasm of a tired attending. In the silence after a student raises a mental health concern. In the praise lavished on those who suffer in stoic silence.

I experienced this hidden curriculum firsthand. Long before a medical board punished me, I was trained to believe that suffering was part of the job. That questioning authority was a sign of arrogance. That the best physicians were the ones who needed the least.

When I faced the fallout of a licensing battle, these lessons came roaring back. I had no road map for advocacy. No language for institutional failure. No training in how to protect myself. My education had prepared me to treat patients, not to survive an unjust system.

This is the danger of the hidden curriculum. It does not prepare physicians for the world they are entering. It prepares them for a world that no longer exists, or perhaps never did.

It assumes a level playing field. It assumes good intentions. It assumes that the system will be fair, that merit will be rewarded, and that excellence will protect you.

None of these assumptions hold.

The modern physician must navigate a world of shifting incentives, opaque and oft-changing regulations, and administrative overreach. They must understand not only medicine but also law, finance, and ethics. And yet, their training still treats these domains as distractions that are irrelevant to the "real" work of taking care of patients.

We need a new curriculum. One that teaches clinical excellence without romanticizing suffering. One that honors vulnerability as a source of strength. One that equips physicians not just to endure, but to lead.

This means teaching business literacy, legal awareness, and emotional intelligence. It means confronting the hidden curriculum and replacing it with a more honest, more humane education.

The MDs we are training today will inherit a system in crisis. And if we do not prepare them for that reality, we are not educating them. We are abandoning them.

CHAPTER 6

The Corporate Takeover of the Physician-Patient Relationship

There was a time when the exam room was a sacred space. It was a place where trust ruled, where expertise mattered, and where decisions were shaped by one thing only: what was best for the patient. For most physicians, that space was the beating heart of their work, the reason they endured the rigors of training, the long nights, and the countless sacrifices. It was the one place where they still felt in control.

That space is disappearing *rapidly.*

Today, physicians find themselves in rooms where their decisions are not fully their own. Invisible hands hover over every interaction: insurance companies, hospital protocols, productivity benchmarks, compliance departments, government guidelines, and pharmaceutical influence. These forces do not enter with stethoscopes or white coats, but they are there nonetheless, shaping what gets said, what gets prescribed, and the kind of care the patient receives.

One of the most powerful of those forces is the pharmaceutical industry. Over the last several decades, it has not only transformed the way Americans consume healthcare but also fundamentally altered the relationship between patients and physicians.

The shift began slowly. In the 1980s and 1990s, drug company representatives became familiar faces in medical offices: friendly, well-dressed, bearing samples, meals, and invitations. At first, the exchanges felt harmless. But over time, the influence deepened. Entire treatment protocols began to evolve around blockbuster drugs. Studies funded by pharmaceutical companies shaped clinical guidelines. Speakers at medical conferences were increasingly revealed to be on company payrolls.

And then came the era of direct-to-consumer advertising.

The moment the US government allowed pharmaceutical companies to market prescription drugs directly to the public, a fundamental shift occurred. No longer did patients rely solely on their physicians for medical guidance. They began to arrive at appointments with drug names in hand, convinced, after seeing an ad on television, that a particular pill was the answer to their suffering. The exam room became a negotiation. The physician's role subtly shifted from advisor to service provider.

This change may seem small, but its implications are enormous. It eroded the trust that once defined medical care. It cast physicians as gatekeepers to a product rather than as partners in the healing process. It commodified health. And for many physicians, it introduced a new kind of pressure: Say yes to keep the patient happy, or say no and risk a complaint, a bad review, or even a loss of income.

This pressure did not come solely from patients. It was reinforced by corporate health systems that began tracking satisfaction scores, prescription rates, and performance data, metrics designed to reflect business priorities more than clinical ones. In this environment, the physician was measured no longer by the quality of care they provided but by how well they conformed to a corporate script.

I felt that shift acutely. In one role, I was expected to meet volume targets that made careful, compassionate care nearly impossible. The system rewarded speed and obedience. When I slowed down to listen more deeply, to teach a patient about lifestyle options instead of reaching for a prescription pad, I found myself reprimanded for inefficiency. Administrators questioned my decisions despite their lack of clinical training. The system expected me to comply, not to think. And when I pushed back, I became a liability.

Some physicians fought back. They refused to overprescribe. They pushed for lifestyle changes when patients wanted pills. They challenged flawed guidelines and raised concerns about overmedicalization. But those who resisted often paid a price: Reputation, support, even employment. Meanwhile, those who complied were rewarded with bonuses, smoother workflows, and approval from systems that had stopped asking whether the care was wise; it only asked whether it was billable.

> *The willingness to do whatever it takes is infinitely more important than knowing everything there is to know about how to do it.*
>
> —Dan S. Kennedy, business expert

Perhaps the most tragic example of this dynamic was the opioid crisis. Fueled by aggressive marketing, supported by misleading data, and driven by perverse incentives, physicians across the country were encouraged—sometimes even coerced—into overprescribing medications that would go on to destroy thousands of lives. Many did so reluctantly, under pressure. Others did so unknowingly, trusting the system that had always claimed to serve science. In both cases, the damage was catastrophic.

That damage wasn't just medical. It was moral. Many physicians emerged from those years feeling betrayed—not only by the industry, but also by their own profession. They began to question everything: the guidelines they had followed, the continuing education they had attended, the research they had relied upon. Some questioned their own role in a system that had profited from pain.

And yet, the machine continued to move forward.

What we see now is not a profession in control of its tools, but a profession surrounded by them, used by them, constrained by them. Pharmaceutical companies shape public perception. Hospitals set financial targets. Insurers determine access. At every turn, the physician must fight to retain even a sliver of clinical autonomy.

The system is not controlled by one hidden hand. It is shaped by many centers of power, each with its own levers of influence. Let's have a quick rundown of ten of them and the countermeasures physicians can use:

1. **Commercial insurers.** They use prior authorization, denials, and all-products clauses. Physicians can respond with payer scorecards, carve-outs, and gold-card campaigns.
2. **Pharmacy benefit managers.** They exclude drugs, demand step therapy, and hide spread pricing. Physicians can respond with transparent PBMs, abandonment tracking, and standard templates.
3. **EHR vendors.** They trap data and create click debt. Physicians can respond with scribe tools, export agreements, and lean dashboards.
4. **Group purchasing organizations.** They bundle products and hide rebates. Physicians can respond with multi-sourcing and physician-led value committees.
5. **Hospital systems.** They control wRVU comp models and referral capture. Physicians can respond with mixed comp plans and open referral networks.
6. **Private equity firms.** They chase EBITDA targets and use non-competes. Physicians can respond with governance protections and quality covenants.
7. **Federal and state payers.** They set fee schedules and flood physicians with measures. Physicians can respond with measure diets, risk accuracy, and collective negotiation.

8. **Accreditation bodies.** They impose costly standards without proven outcomes. Physicians can respond by demanding evidence and aligning policies with real risks.
9. **Malpractice insurers.** They set premiums and push settlements. Physicians can respond with documentation playbooks and early disclosure protocols.
10. **Big Tech and retail disruptors.** They control data and patient funnels. Physicians can respond with transparent pricing, local referral networks, and API rights.

These are not abstract problems. They are daily pressures that shape how physicians practice and how patients are treated. When you name them clearly, you can finally push back.

Some of the most exhausting aspects of modern medical practice are not clinical, but bureaucratic. What used to be time spent with patients is now devoured by checkboxes, portals, authorizations, and data entry. Even a routine prescription can require lengthy justification, additional approvals, and the navigation of shifting insurance formularies. Physicians often find themselves doing more documentation than diagnosis. Many spend hours after clinic notes are closed, not reviewing labs or thinking through patient care, but cleaning up digital records so they can bill properly. The consequences are not just emotional. They are structural. Hospitals and corporations set the rules, and physicians must comply or risk losing access to platforms, payment, or positions.

Prior authorization is the clearest example. It blocks timely care and erodes trust. But it can be managed with structure.

1. **Gold card pursuit.** Exempt physicians with a strong record of appropriate use.
2. **Single-touch rule.** Submit a complete standards-based package the first time.
3. **Escalation ladder.** Advance each case on a timed path from nurse to physician to medical director.

4. **Peer-to-peer library.** Share the winning arguments across service lines.
5. **Denial analytics.** Track what gets denied and fix the root cause.

This is not about gaming a system. It is about restoring access to necessary care and giving physicians the time to practice medicine.

Burnout has become so widespread not only because of what physicians face in their day, but also because of how little control they have over any of it. The term *moral injury* has begun to replace *burnout* for good reason. Physicians are not just tired. They are forced to participate in care that contradicts their training and their ethics. Many feel they have become cogs in a machine that does not value their voice or trust their judgment. This quiet despair is one of the profession's most urgent crises. It is not rooted in weakness. It is rooted in systems that profit from physician compliance but rarely invest in their restoration.

What gets lost in all of this is the patient. Not the patient as a consumer. Not the patient's satisfaction score. But the human being who walks into a room vulnerable, confused, and in need of someone they can trust. The physician is still that person—still the one with the knowledge, the training, the heart to help. But the physician's hands are increasingly tied.

This is not the fault of individual physicians. It is the result of a system that has slowly redefined what medicine is. A system that has transformed healthcare from a relationship into a transaction. That has replaced ethical judgment with algorithmic oversight. And that has convinced the public that more treatment, more drugs, more branding equals better care.

The physicians who resist this transformation, who still see their work as sacred, are often the ones who suffer most. They feel out of step. Alone. Angry. Some burn out. Others quit. A few try to build something different.

But the fight is not theirs alone. If we are to reclaim medicine as a profession of healing and truth, we must name what has happened. We must be willing to say that the physician-patient relationship has been hijacked. This has not been done by malice but by momentum. Not by a single villain but by a system that rewards obedience and punishes integrity.

It is not too late to recover what has been lost. However, it will require courage, not just from physicians but also from institutions, educators, and patients themselves. We must be willing to listen again to the people in the white coats—not the ones on the bill-boards or in the boardrooms, but the ones still trying, every day, to make medicine human again.

CHAPTER 7

The Productivity Trap

One of the most insidious changes in modern medicine is the quiet transformation of the physician from a healer into a producer. Not a producer of health or wellness, but of volume: patient visits, billable codes, relative value units. Somewhere along the way, the quality of a physician's work stopped being measured by its depth and began to be measured by its speed.

This shift did not happen all at once. It crept in through administrative pressure, reimbursement models, and the increasing corporatization of healthcare. At first, it looked like optimization. Then it became normalization. Today, it is simply the expectation: more patients per hour, more documentation, more throughput. Less time to think. Less time to care. More overtime paperwork.

For physicians, the consequences are profound. Productivity targets result in shorter visits and faster decision-making. They mean less time for complexity, conversation, and connection. They mean more pressure to defer to algorithms, template notes, and checklists designed for compliance rather than understanding.

I lived that reality. In one of my positions, my schedule was filled to capacity every day, without regard for the nuance or needs of the patients I served. I was praised for efficiency when I hit benchmarks, but reprimanded when I took the time necessary for care that was truly comprehensive. I began to feel like a machine—one expected to diagnose, treat, and chart with the speed of automation, but with none of the support or humanity that meaningful medicine requires.

It was not the medicine that wore me down. It was the machinery around it. The sense that my value had been reduced to the number of patients I could move through a system that seemed to prize volume over value. I had once imagined medicine as a profession of deep listening and careful thought. What I encountered instead was a conveyor belt.

> *All businesses succeed or die depending on the effectiveness of their marketing systems.*
>
> —Dan S. Kennedy, business expert

This is what physicians mean when they say the work has changed. It is not that patients are more difficult. It is that the system gives them less time, fewer tools, and little support to meet those difficulties well. Physicians are being asked to do more with less, and then blamed for not doing it fast enough.

In such an environment, moral injury becomes common. Physicians are forced to choose between what they know is right and what the system demands. They carry the weight of decisions made under duress. They feel the sting of being measured not by the care they provide, but by how well they conform to artificial standards.

Some institutions try to respond with wellness programs. But no amount of yoga or mindfulness will fix a system that punishes thoughtfulness and rewards haste. What physicians need is not stress relief. They need structural relief. They need workflows designed around care, not around quotas.

Reclaiming medicine from the productivity trap will not be easy. It will require courage from leadership, honesty from policymakers, and sustained advocacy from physicians themselves. But the alternative is clear. If we do not change how we measure success in medicine, we will continue to lose the very people we need to deliver it.

Physicians are not asking for less work. They are asking for meaningful work. They are asking to be seen as professionals, not producers. They are asking for a system that values what they offer—not just their time, but their judgment, their integrity, and their humanity.

If we want a healthcare system that truly serves patients, we must first build one that respects the people trying to care for them. That means ending the reign of productivity as the primary metric. It means building space for complexity, for conversation, for care that takes the time it needs. Only then can medicine become what it was always meant to be: not a race against the clock, but a relationship built on trust.

Part 2
The Human Cost

CHAPTER 8

THE UNSEEN STAKEHOLDERS

When discussing the crisis in American medicine, we often focus the conversation on physicians and patients. But there is another group that must be addressed. It includes those who help shape, administer, and influence the systems that govern medical practice. These stakeholders include hospital administrators, insurance executives, medical board members, state and federal regulators, and many others whose decisions impact daily medical life.

For lasting reform to take root, these stakeholders must not only be engaged, but also held to a higher standard of accountability and purpose. After all, their decisions, made in conference rooms and courtrooms, have real consequences for the people on the ground.

Too often, these non-physician stakeholders hold immense sway over the trajectory of a physician's career without the necessary insight into what it means to practice medicine. Medical boards, for example, include non-physician appointees who often vote on the fate of physicians brought before them. These individuals may lack the clinical expertise or nuanced understanding necessary to make fair assessments of complex medical decisions.

Accountability is essential, but it must be informed. If non-physicians are to serve on boards with the power to end medical careers, they must be educated about the complexity of medical decision-making. If hospital leaders and payers are to mandate productivity standards, they must be willing to listen to those affected. If regulators and legislators are to pass laws that affect patient care, they must include physicians in meaningful consultation.

No system can survive when the people making the rules are insulated from the reality of those who live by them. That is why stakeholder reform must be a central part of any solution.

We must elevate the expectations we place on non-physician influencers. We must redefine their roles not simply as watchdogs or bureaucrats, but as partners in the preservation of a profession that still holds the power to heal. Reform is not only about giving physicians a voice. It is also about ensuring that everyone who speaks into the profession is worthy of being heard.

CHAPTER 9

The Training That Teaches Silence

For most physicians, the story of their professional life begins not with their first job but with their first day of medical school. It is there, in the lecture halls and anatomy labs, that they begin to absorb not only the science of medicine but also the culture that surrounds it. And that culture is what leaves the most profound imprint.

From the beginning, medical training is a study in endurance. Students are taught to memorize vast amounts of information, perform under pressure, and accept grueling hours without complaint. The system rewards perfectionism and punishes vulnerability. Mistakes are framed not as opportunities to grow but as signs of weakness. Emotional expression is rarely encouraged. Doubt is often silenced. And self-sacrifice is valorized above all.

I remember this culture well. Early in my training, I was praised for my discipline and dedication. I did not question the demands placed on me. When I felt overwhelmed, I pushed through. When I encountered moments of ethical discomfort and times when a patient's needs clashed with administrative demands, I suppressed the urge to speak out. That silence wasn't cowardice. It was learned.

I once had a rotation during which a senior resident reprimanded a patient who didn't understand the discharge instructions. Everything in me wanted to intervene. But I didn't. I told myself I didn't want to step out of line, didn't want to compromise my evaluations. I carried that silence with me for years.

That moment was just one of many. Over time, I, like many physicians, internalized the lesson: Survive first, speak later. But later, it turned out, rarely came. What starts as a temporary coping strategy often becomes a permanent habit.

This silent conditioning persists even after graduation. It follows physicians into practice, shaping how they respond to unsafe workloads, unethical policies, or unjust treatment. It explains why so many physicians suffer in isolation, afraid to admit what they're feeling until it's too late.

The cost of that silence is enormous. It prevents honest conversations about burnout, workplace trauma, and systemic injustice. It reinforces a culture in which suffering is normalized and seeking help is viewed as a sign of weakness rather than a form of strength. And it leads many to walk away not just from a job but from a calling that once felt sacred.

Medical education must change. It must teach not only clinical excellence but also emotional resilience, ethical courage, and professional boundaries. It must normalize discomfort, encourage dialogue, and make space for the full humanity of the people who choose this path.

That change begins with naming the truth: We have built a system that conditions silence, and we are paying the price for it.

If we want physicians to speak up when something is wrong, we must first teach them that their voice matters. If we want them to lead, we must stop training them to fade into the background.

I finally found my voice again, but only after significant cost. Others may not be as fortunate. We owe it to the next generation to give them a different starting point. Not one defined by silence, but one defined by the courage to speak, the strength to question, and the freedom to care without fear.

CHAPTER 10

When Physicians Have No Voice

In any profession, accountability matters. But in medicine, the stakes are uniquely high. Decisions are made in real time, often under intense pressure, and lives hang in the balance. When a physician makes a mistake, or is even accused of one, the consequences can be profound. It is essential that systems of oversight exist. But oversight, without fairness, becomes persecution. And when physicians are denied a voice in their own defense, the entire profession suffers.

I know this firsthand. I had built a successful OB/GYN practice and, like many responsible physicians, had secured multiple state licenses early in my career to allow for future mobility. It was a strategic move, based on sound reasoning and the realities of medical practice. But that preparation could not protect me from what came next.

I applied for a license in Arizona, thinking it would be a routine process. I had no pending issues. I wasn't under investigation. I just wanted to keep my options open. I went to the board meeting alone. I didn't think I needed a lawyer. That was my first mistake.

During the meeting, a past case was raised. It was the one I talked about earlier in this book. It was a complicated delivery involving a patient who had explicitly refused a C-section. I had managed the labor carefully, remained at the bedside, and delivered the child without any complications at the time. But one physician on the board (one possibly not even trained in OB/GYN) launched into a ten-minute tirade against me. The other board members followed suit. I wasn't allowed to respond.

I sat there, completely stunned. I had spent nearly 20 years delivering babies, managing complex cases, and mentoring younger physicians. And none of that mattered in that room. They judged me based on a single case, filtered through one person's outrage.

The board denied my license.

The experience was not just personally devastating; it was professionally destabilizing. destabilizing. And it didn't end there. The Arizona board's decision was quietly shared with other states. Soon, California took up the same case. But this time, there wasn't even a hearing with the board. I was summoned to appear before a local court.

I thought it would be a conversation. It wasn't. It was a courtroom. No jury. No medical experts. There was just a judge (who I later learned was in the middle of a hostile divorce from her OB/GYN husband). That bias colored everything. She wasn't interested in the facts. She didn't want to hear my side.

The result? A suspension of my license. A demand that I repeat my entire residency if I wanted to continue practicing OB. It was, in effect, a career-ending sentence.

The cumulative impact of these proceedings was catastrophic. I was blackballed from malpractice insurance across the country. No practice. No income. No future in my specialty.

I had three kids. A wife. No way to support them. And no appeal. I remember sitting in my car, wondering if it was worth going on. But something in me refused to quit. Maybe it was the fighter in me from my days in Vietnam. Maybe it was God. But I knew I had to find another path.

What Happens When the Board Comes for You

They don't tell you this part in medical school. Over the course of their career, around 25 percent of physicians will face a state medical board investigation at least once.

They don't prepare you for what it means to have the state turn its full bureaucratic attention toward you. By the time a medical board brings down a judgment, the most painful part is often not the formal punishment. It's the slow unraveling of your career and identity in the months and years that follow.

The punishment doesn't just stop at a license restriction. It metastasizes. It infects everything.

You Are Marked

Once you've been disciplined, your name is entered into the National Practitioner Data Bank. This isn't some dusty government filing cabinet. It's a public database that anyone can search. Patients. Hospitals. Insurance carriers. Attorneys. They all get access to it.

And they will use it.

One mark, even if it was based on a philosophical disagreement or a documentation issue, becomes your calling card in every interview, application, or referral network from that point forward.

Doors Close Quietly

The job you held may vanish overnight. Hospital credentials get pulled. Referrals dry up. Insurance companies cancel your malpractice coverage or hike your premiums so high it amounts to the same thing. New job applications are either stalled or denied without explanation.

Suddenly, the work you trained for decades to do becomes unavailable to you. The opportunities shrink. Some physicians are pushed into early retirement. Others take jobs in remote or underserved areas, where the hiring bar is lower and the scrutiny thinner. It is not a transfer. It's an exile, one compounded by a lack of business education when they seek non-medical practice jobs.

You Lose More Than a License

What stings most is not the job loss. It's the identity loss.

We are trained to believe that being a doctor is not just what we do, but who we are. When that identity is attacked or stripped away, it does something to you. I've seen colleagues descend into depression, isolation, even addiction. Some of them never recover.

And if you think the profession will rally around you, you're mistaken. Most colleagues, even those who know better, keep their distance. You are treated like you're contagious.

There Is No Way Back

You'd think there would be some kind of formal path for restoration, a way that lets a physician demonstrate growth, learning, or change. But no such path exists.

You are excluded from publications. Removed from medical society leadership. Forbidden from speaking at conferences or mentoring residents. The medical establishment does not offer a way back. The damage is permanent.

And the Worst Part? You Might Have Been Right

Many of the doctors who are sanctioned are not charlatans or quacks. They are physicians who practiced with courage. Who refused to follow the herd. Who treated patients as individuals instead of protocols.

Their only crime was offering care that didn't conform to the narrow and shifting expectations of a medical bureaucracy increasingly influenced by non-medical interests. That's the part that breaks your heart. And it should make you angry.

I eventually found a way to practice again, supported by a hospital that covered my malpractice insurance and a state willing to issue a license. But the scars remain. And my story is not unique.

Medical boards were created to protect the public. But too often, they punish physicians without fairness or context. Here are the most common failure points:

- Specialty mismatches where reviewers lack expertise. Board members, especially physicians, are not skilled in the specialty training of the person brought before them, so they cannot understand the nuances of the medical situation.
- Public members who vote on clinical issues without training.
- Vague evidentiary standards that ignore guidelines. As one example, the standard in OB/GYN is that after the patient pushes for two hours, a C-section is recommended. This standard would result in an unnecessary increase in C-sections by thousands for mothers who would otherwise give birth naturally and with no problems if more time were given.
- Processes that move faster for the board than for the physician.
- Conflicts of interest and biases that are never disclosed.

These failures do not just harm individual physicians. They weaken the trust that allows medicine to function at all. The solution begins with due process. Here are the rights every physician should be guaranteed:

1. Specialty-matched peer review by at least two experts in the same specialty.
2. Evidence standards that cite guidelines and record minority opinions.
3. Public members trained and limited to ethical or behavioral review.
4. Access to case files with defined timelines for response.
5. Independent hearing examiners, not board members, for disputed facts.
6. Written conflict disclosures with the right to challenge reviewers.

7. Graduated remedies that use education first when harm is not proven.
8. Published and anonymized decisions to create precedent.

Without these rights, justice is impossible. With them, the profession has a chance to recover its integrity.

State medical boards are essential. But they must be fair, transparent, and rooted in due process. When decisions are made behind closed doors, without complete information, and with no opportunity for defense, they cease to serve the public good. They become tools of destruction.

Physicians deserve accountability, but they also deserve justice. They deserve a chance to explain, to clarify, to learn, and, when appropriate, to recover.

My experience reveals a deeper problem in our system: a willingness to discard dedicated physicians based on incomplete narratives and unchecked authority. We cannot afford to lose more good physicians to silence, shame, or systemic failure.

The silence we face is not only in courtrooms or board meetings. It also exists in day-to-day clinical life, where physicians are rarely invited to shape the policies that govern their work. Decisions about workflow, reimbursement, documentation, and care delivery are often made without their input. Those who try to speak up are dismissed or labeled as difficult. Those who comply are rewarded with temporary security but must carry the internal weight of knowing they had no voice.

This erosion of influence begins early. Medical students are trained to follow, not to challenge. Residents are rewarded for endurance, not inquiry. By the time physicians reach independent practice, many have internalized the idea that their role is to implement rather than to lead. And when they do speak, they are met with systems designed to absorb complaints without ever shifting direction.

But physicians are not interchangeable cogs. They are trained thinkers, moral agents, and skilled observers of human life. When their voice is muted, the entire system loses access to one of its most valuable sources of wisdom. That loss is not theoretical. It shows up in poorly designed workflows, in misguided policy, in rising burnout, and in worsening patient outcomes.

We must protect the integrity of medicine, not only by holding physicians accountable, but also by ensuring that the systems designed to do so are just, humane, and grounded in truth and scientific research or data.

CHAPTER 11

When the System Profits from Silence

Medicine has always demanded resilience. Long hours, difficult conversations, and the weight of human vulnerability are part of the calling. But what happens when that resilience is not enough to shield physicians from the harms inflicted by the very system they serve?

I faced that question in the quiet aftermath of a disciplinary ruling. The impact of losing my license and being effectively blackballed from the profession I had spent decades practicing was more than logistical. It was psychological. For a time, I lived in silence, carrying the burden alone.

I was afraid to talk about what had happened. Not just because of shame, but because of fear. Fear that if I spoke openly, I would be seen as bitter or disgraced. Fear that I would never work again. That fear is not unique to me. It is something countless physicians carry.

I remember how isolating it felt to go from being a respected colleague and teacher to someone people whispered about. I remember how the silence around my story made me question not just my career, but my worth too. I didn't know where to go. I didn't know who to trust. And most painfully, I didn't know if my story even mattered.

This is the hidden cost of a system that punishes physicians without space for redemption. It creates a culture where physicians cannot speak openly about hardship, injustice, or trauma. Where a single judgment can erase decades of contribution. And where silence becomes a survival strategy.

We must make space for these stories, not to excuse harm, but to understand it. To learn. To rebuild. To prevent the same pain from happening to others.

I eventually found my voice again. I began to tell the truth about what happened. And in doing so, I discovered I was not alone. Other physicians began to reach out. Some had been disciplined unfairly. Others had walked away from the profession under similar clouds. Some had lost their practices, their health, their sense of self.

These stories are not rare. They are simply hidden. Buried under the pressure to appear unshakable. Left out of the narrative we tell about what it means to be a physician.

> *Today's medical schools typically provide minimal instruction about the business of medicine and the way healthcare systems work, but future physicians must be well versed in these topics so they can thrive in rapidly changing settings.*
>
> —Ardis D. Hoven, MD

Physician silence benefits no one except the systems that profit from keeping physicians compliant and quiet. When physicians are afraid to speak, reform becomes impossible. When they are isolated, innovation dies. When they are shamed into submission, medicine itself becomes brittle.

The Medical Deep State isn't about healing. Rather, it is focused on managing perception. It convinces the public that the institutions in power care, while continuing to grind its workforce into dust. It is time to create a culture that honors transparency. That allows physicians to speak honestly about their experiences without fear of retaliation. That not only welcomes accountability but also offers compassion.

I hope that my story reminds us that healing isn't just for patients. It must also be for the healers. And that sometimes, the bravest thing a physician can do is tell the truth, even when the system prefers silence.

CHAPTER 12

The Consequences of Being Conditioned to Endure

Our future is preordained by our past unless we intervene in the present.

—Dan S. Kennedy, business expert

In medicine, endurance is a badge of honor. From their earliest days of training, physicians are taught to push through exhaustion, suppress emotions, and keep going even when every signal in their body and mind tells them otherwise. This conditioning is not subtle. It is built into the structure of education and residency. Mentors, rewarded by institutions, reinforce it and are rarely questioned.

I remember those lessons clearly. Call nights when sleep was a luxury. Hours spent standing in surgeries after already working a full day. The culture of never showing weakness, never saying no, never admitting when the weight was too much. That pattern didn't stop when I finished training. It simply evolved.

I was proud of being able to take it. Of doing what others wouldn't. I was proud of never missing a delivery, never leaving my patients hanging. But somewhere along the way, that pride became a trap. The system didn't care how much I gave; it only noticed if I stopped.

That mindset led me to say yes when I should have said no. To accept more patients, more hours, more responsibility. It wasn't just work ethic. It was identity. And it nearly broke me.

I'm not alone. Across the profession, physicians are paying a high price for a culture that equates worth with overwork. They delay care for their own illnesses. They suppress symptoms of depression, anxiety, and burnout. They ignore red flags because stopping feels like failure.

But the consequences are real. Relationships suffer. Mental health deteriorates. Mistakes happen. Some MDs walk away. Others die by suicide. And many simply fade. They remain present but hollowed out, going through the motions in a profession that once gave them life.

The system reinforces this pattern by rewarding compliance and punishing those who set boundaries. Physicians who set limits are seen as less committed. Those who ask for support are viewed with suspicion. And those who leave are often forgotten.

My story highlights a painful irony: The very qualities that make great physicians—dedication, endurance, and self-sacrifice—are the same ones that the system exploits. And when we fall, there is rarely a safety net.

We must reimagine what it means to be a committed physician. It cannot mean endless giving without replenishment. It cannot mean silence in the face of harm. It must include sustainability, self-awareness, and the freedom to ask for help.

That starts with training. It starts with reshaping the culture of medical education to normalize rest, reflection, and recovery. It continues in practice, where institutions must protect time, respect limits, and view physicians not as resources to be maximized but as human beings to be supported.

I learned, too late, that endurance without care becomes self-destruction. My journey back from collapse to clarity was long and hard. But it gave me something rare in medicine: the perspective to question the culture, and the courage to tell the truth about it.

That truth is this: Endurance is not the goal. Health is. And until we teach physicians to care for themselves with the same urgency they bring to their patients, we will continue to lose them—quietly, tragically, and unnecessarily.

CHAPTER 13

The Disillusionment of a Calling

You have absolute control over but one thing: your thoughts. This divine prerogative is the sole means by which you may control your destiny. If you fail to control your mind, you will control nothing else. Your mind is your spiritual estate. What you hold in your mind today will shape your experiences of tomorrow.

—Napoleon Hill, author of Think and Grow Rich

For many, medicine begins as a calling. It's not just a career path; it's a moral undertaking. Aspiring physicians enter the profession with a deep sense of purpose, shaped by idealism and a desire to make a meaningful difference. But that calling can be tested, stretched, and sometimes broken by the realities of modern practice.

I carried that calling with me from the very beginning. I didn't just want to be a physician. I felt born to it. The science excited me, but the human connection—the chance to be present at the most vulnerable and transformative moments of people's lives—was what truly moved me. I thought that dedication would be enough. That if I showed up, worked hard, and stayed true to the oath I had taken, the system would support me.

It didn't.

I believed medicine was sacred. That belief carried me through training, through sleepless nights, through moments of doubt. But once I was out in the real world, it felt like every part of the system was working against the care I wanted to provide. The time pressures, administrative hurdles, and corporate protocols kept me feeling as if I were constantly being pulled away from the patient, which was the entire reason I was there in the first place.

Over time, that distance turned into disillusionment. I didn't lose my love for medicine. I lost my trust in the system that claimed to support it. I began to question whether the calling that had once felt so pure had a place in a structure that prioritized volume over value, metrics over meaning.

I am far from alone.

Every time a physician tells the truth about what's happening, the Medical Deep State moves to protect itself. It does not welcome transparency. It sees it as a threat.

Across the country, physicians are wrestling with this same dissonance. They came to heal, to comfort, to lead. But they are increasingly reduced to cogs in a machine they didn't design and can't fully influence. The pressures of productivity quotas, risk management protocols, and EMR checkboxes crowd out the space for curiosity, reflection, and presence.

The result is not just frustration. It is moral injury, which is the distress that arises when professionals are forced to act in ways that contradict their core values. When physicians are told to discharge a patient before they're ready, to withhold care due to insurance constraints, to ignore what their clinical intuition tells them because a policy says otherwise, they don't just feel constrained. They feel complicit.

And that feeling is corrosive. Disillusionment in medicine doesn't mean physicians no longer care. It means they care so much that the system's indifference becomes unbearable. It means they're still trying to honor the calling that led them here, even as it becomes harder to bear.

We can't rebuild trust without acknowledging this breach. We can't call medicine a calling while expecting its practitioners to practice in ways that betray their values.

Restoring that sense of purpose starts with listening to the physicians whose voices have been muted by bureaucracy and burnout. It means reforming the structures that corrode their integrity. And it means reimagining leadership so that those who still believe in the sacredness of the work have the power to protect it.

I haven't abandoned my calling. But I've had to redefine it on my own terms. What once felt like a straight path now feels more like a daily choice: To stay grounded, to stay human, and to stay in the fight for a kind of medicine that still deserves the name.

If we want others to make that choice, we have to give them a reason to believe it's worth it.

CHAPTER 14

When There Are No Physicians Left

There are lessons we carry from moments that never leave us. I was serving as a Flight Surgeon for a Marine Helicopter Squadron in Vietnam when an Army Special Forces physician approached me with an invitation. His unit was planning a "Village Sick Call," and he asked if I would join them. I said yes without hesitation. My work rarely gave me the chance to meet Vietnamese civilians, and I wanted that opportunity.

The next morning, I climbed into the back of one of five military trucks, not knowing what awaited us. The village lay about eight to ten miles outside Da Nang, along dusty roads lined with people on foot. As we rode, I was briefed on the rules: the fifteen Special Forces soldiers would take up guard positions while we worked in the open, treating whoever came forward. It was dangerous ground. Teenage boys and men often worked the rice fields by day, then fought with the Viet Cong at night.

When we arrived, I noticed immediately that no young men were in sight. Instead, a line stretched before us made up of women, children, and elderly men. The Viet Cong were likely nearby, watching, but we were left alone. Later I would learn why: They valued the medications we handed out far more than the chance to kill us. After we left, they would simply collect the pills from the villagers and keep them for themselves.

Through Vietnamese interpreters, the two of us physicians saw patient after patient. We handed out what little we could, often just a pill or two. There were times when I saw things that shook me, like a tumor protruding from an old man's body, for instance, but I was forbidden from doing more. No biopsies. No referrals. Not even a stethoscope against a chest. Just a pill and a nod.

I discovered that South Vietnam had only 600 physicians. They were all located in Saigon, the capital. There were no physicians available anywhere else. Most patients had to travel hundreds of miles to see a doctor. This situation could eventually happen in the United States as well, due to physician attrition, unless we begin to import doctors from outside the country. Such an outcome would affect healthcare negatively, as they will bring their own medical perspectives and practices that conflict with our cultural norms.

Near the end of the day, a middle-aged woman stepped forward, keeping her son close behind her. When the boy finally emerged, I saw the extent of his injuries. He had been burned by white phosphorus from our own bombs. His right arm and hand were fused tightly to his side by thick scars. He had no use of them.

The mother looked at me with desperate eyes. Through the interpreter, I told her what I thought. I told her that with surgery, the scars could be cut away, and her boy might one day move his arm and hand again. When she heard this, she began to cry. So did I. She had never imagined such a thing was possible.

I arranged for the boy to be sent for surgical treatment, though I never learned if it happened. I doubt it did. But I will never forget the moment when that mother realized, for the first time, that her son's life might not be as limited as she had believed.

That day showed me two things I have never forgotten. First, that people carry unbearable burdens silently, until hope is offered. And second, that when physicians are present, available, and empowered to act, they become the thin line between despair and possibility.

Today, I fear we are approaching a civilian version of that powerless day in the village. A patient will walk into a clinic or emergency room and be told, "There is no physician available." Not because of war or geography, but because of bureaucratic indifference. Because the system has slowly dismantled what used to be the physician's rightful place at the center of care in our nation.

This is not some distant, foreign possibility. It is happening in rural communities already. It is showing up in emergency rooms that are stretched too thin. And it will become commonplace if we continue to undermine the viability of private practice, suppress physician leadership, and reduce doctors to interchangeable providers in systems they no longer control.

The system is cracking. We can hear it if we choose to listen. Physician burnout is not just an HR problem. It is a public warning. The collapse of independent practice is not just an economic event. It is a signal that the last line of personalized, community-based care is under siege.

When there are no physicians left, society will not simply miss their technical skills. We will miss their judgment, their advocacy, their deep knowledge of a patient's history, and their ability to spot something that cannot be explained by a checkbox in an EHR. We will be left with protocols instead of discernment, metrics instead of meaning, and systems that work for no one.

The time to turn this around is now. Not later. Not after the next round of hospital consolidations. Not after one more policy report. We already know what happens when no one is available to respond. I have seen it. And so have others. If we fail to act, our children and grandchildren will one day walk into a hospital and be told that a physician is no longer part of the care team. They will be told to wait, or be referred elsewhere, or be treated by a system that does not know their name.

We cannot let that be the legacy of this generation. We must restore the place of the physician in the center of care. We must act while there is still time.

Some argue the answer is to import more physicians from abroad. That may help, but it cannot replace the urgent need to keep the physicians we already have. Both matter. We must

- Fix the system so current physicians can and want to stay.
- Streamline entry for qualified international physicians who meet the same standards.

We cannot build a sustainable system by losing our own physicians faster than we train new ones. Retention must come first. Expansion can follow, but only with the same high standards for everyone.

Part 3
Stakeholder Conversations

CHAPTER 15

To Hospital and Health System Leaders: Partner with Physicians, or Lose Them

You may not wear the white coat. You may not write prescriptions or deliver bad news to families at 3 a.m. But make no mistake: you hold enormous influence over what modern medicine feels like for MDs, for patients, and for entire communities.

And right now, many of the physicians in your system feel like they're suffocating under your leadership.

It didn't start with evil intent. You stepped in during times of growth, of crisis, of complexity. You brought operational acumen, business discipline, and systems thinking. You helped stabilize institutions, drive quality improvement, and streamline processes that had become dangerously fragmented. These contributions matter.

However, somewhere along the way, a more profound imbalance began to take hold. Physicians became employees. Metrics replaced trust. Productivity targets drowned out professional judgment. And decisions about care began to be made farther and farther from the bedside.

Now, your physicians are burning out in record numbers. Things are turning more and more toward telehealth. They are retiring early, reducing their hours, or leaving the medical field altogether. And many of them are not leaving because of the work itself. They are leaving because of you.

I felt this shift long before I had the language to describe it. I recall the moment I realized the culture of my hospital had shifted. I was still doing the same work, but everything around me felt heavier. It wasn't just the pace or the charting. It was the fact that every decision seemed to be second-guessed by someone who wasn't in the room.

I had always believed in collaboration. I welcomed oversight when it served the safety and quality of the product. But I could feel the slow erosion of autonomy. It was the way clinical judgment was replaced with flowcharts and care pathways became rigid protocols.

I started to dread meetings, not because of the work, but because I knew that nothing I said would really make a difference. I was on committees, but not in a position of power. I was asked for input, but never for a vote. Eventually, I stopped volunteering. What was the point?

Hospitals do not heal people. People heal people.

And when the people doing the healing feel devalued, surveilled, and silenced, your system may survive on paper, but the soul of it is gone. Culture erodes in quiet ways: through ignored feedback, unrewarded sacrifice, and the unspoken message that physicians are labor, not leaders.

You have the power to change this, not by stepping out of the room, but by bringing physicians back into it.

Bring them into the rooms where strategy is set, where staffing ratios are determined, and where budgets are established. Stop appointing physician leaders as figureheads to manage optics. Start empowering them as full partners. Give them actual decision rights. Real resources. Protected time.

If your physicians only feel heard when there's a crisis, they're not heard. If your staff surveys go unread or get buried beneath benchmark comparisons, you're not listening. If your EMR optimization efforts are led by people who've never charted a 12-hour shift, you're not solving the right problem.

Eventually, I left hospital employment. I didn't leave because I couldn't do the work. I left because I felt invisible. Replaceable. Like everything I brought to the table—years of training, hard-won intuition, deep relationships with patients—meant less than a line on a spreadsheet.

You may believe that you've done everything you can. The labor market is tight. That budgets are constrained. That change is hard. All of that may be true. However, until you change how you treat your physicians by respecting them as thinkers, as leaders, and as the cornerstone of your mission, you are simply managing decline.

And decline is what's coming if you do nothing. Physician shortages are growing. Patient trust is fraying. The generational pipeline is thinning. Younger MDs are not willing to endure what their mentors did, and they shouldn't have to.

They want flexibility. Respect. A say in how care is delivered. They want to be measured by outcomes, not RVUs. They want to innovate, not just execute. And they want to believe that if they give their best years to your institution, they won't be discarded when the budget tightens.

You do not need to be perfect. But you do need to be honest.

If you believe physicians matter, then build structures that reflect that belief. If you believe patient care is sacred, then protect the people who deliver it. If you believe in long-term value, stop treating your workforce like a short-term line item.

Trust is not a line in a mission statement. It's built into how you allocate time, power, and attention.

Reimagine the way you lead. Build co-governance models. Invest in physician development, not just compliance training. Align incentives with mission, not just margin. Remove punitive productivity models that punish reflection, teaching, or complexity. Allow dissent to be voiced without retaliation. Celebrate courage, not just efficiency.

If you're unsure what your physicians really need, ask them. And then act on what you hear.

Because if you don't act, you won't just lose your workforce. You'll lose your edge. Your reputation. Your ability to attract and keep people who could choose to work elsewhere, or not at all.

You can still lead. But only if you redefine what leadership means.

Not command and control. Not more metrics. Not another consulting firm. What medicine needs now are leaders who understand that care cannot be standardized into a one-size-fits-all approach. That quality cannot be manufactured without dignity. And that healing begins with those who deliver it feeling whole themselves.

Partner with physicians. Share power. Let them help you lead. Or keep managing the fallout of a workforce that is slipping through your fingers, one silent resignation at a time.

CHAPTER 16

To Policymakers and Regulators: Regulate with, Not over, Physicians

You write the rules. You shape the incentives. You craft the guardrails that define the boundaries of modern medicine.

And in doing so, you hold forms of power that physicians cannot match: legislative, procedural, and systemic. You determine how healthcare is reimbursed, how it is monitored, and in many ways, how it is experienced by physicians and patients alike.

But too often, that power is wielded without the one thing it needs most: proximity to the people doing the work.

It is easy to believe that if a law or rule serves the public interest in theory, it must be doing good in practice. But in medicine, intent and impact often diverge. Policies that look clean on paper can create chaos at the bedside. And when the physician's voice is absent from policymaking, unintended consequences become the norm.

Physicians are not against regulation. We understand the need for oversight, for safety standards, for ethical boundaries. What we are asking for is not the removal of rules. It is the right to help shape them.

Too many of today's regulations are written by individuals who have never practiced medicine, and are enforced by systems that assume compliance is equivalent to quality. But care is not a code to be followed. It is a relationship to be protected. And rules that ignore that truth, however well-intended, end up pushing physicians out of the profession we love.

The irony is painful. We are losing some of the best-trained minds in the country, not because they failed to keep up, but because the system won't let them slow down. We are regulating the very soul out of medicine.

You have the power to reverse this. To pause. To listen. To involve physicians not as occasional advisors, but as co-authors of policy. To conduct human impact audits of healthcare legislation. To ask not just "What problem are we solving?" but also "At what cost, and to whom?"

What would change if every new regulation required a review by a panel of practicing physicians? If policy proposals had to be piloted in real-world settings before full implementation? If reimbursement formulas were crafted with the input of frontline clinicians who understand both the numbers and the nuance?

What would change if scope-of-practice debates were guided not just by workforce economics, but by clinical realities and patient safety? If licensure rules supported mobility and innovation instead of punishing complexity?

We know the pressures you face. The budget constraints. The lobbying noise. The headlines that demand quick fixes. However, real reform requires more than just urgency. It takes alignment. And alignment only happens when you see physicians as collaborators, not just constituents.

You don't have to fix everything. However, you must stop causing harm in the name of helping.

Start by simplifying what you can. Streamline reporting requirements. Align metrics across programs. Reduce redundant audits.

Protect physicians from legal and financial threats that discourage risk-taking, especially in underserved communities.

And above all, stop writing policies that assume physicians are the problem. Start writing policies that enable us to be the solution.

You have an extraordinary opportunity. You can be the generation of lawmakers and regulators who helped save the medical profession from further collapse, not by writing more rules, but by writing better ones.

Rules that are shaped in partnership. Incentives that reward depth, not just volume. Metrics that track outcomes, not just throughput. And structures that support the kind of care you'd want for your own family.

This is how the Medical Deep State operates. Not with overt threats, but with quiet removal of privilege. With investigations that drag on. With whispers behind closed doors that label good doctors as dangerous.

We are not asking for special treatment. We are asking for sanity. For respect. For a chance to practice with the freedom and integrity our training demands.

Give us that chance, not just because it is good politics, but because it is the only way that healthcare becomes what it was always meant to be: not a system of compliance, but a culture of care.

CHAPTER 17

To Medical Educators: Teach More Than Science

You shape the beginning. You decide what gets taught, what gets prioritized, and what gets internalized by the next generation of physicians. You are the stewards of medicine's moral and intellectual foundation. And right now, that foundation, outdated by decades, is cracking.

We ask medical students to memorize impossible volumes of information, to perform under extreme pressure, and to adopt an identity of quiet endurance. We teach them anatomy, pathology, pharmacology, and physiology. But we do not teach them how to protect themselves. We do not teach them how to lead.

We tell students that medicine is a calling, but we don't prepare them for what it means to answer that call in a broken system. We don't teach them about contracts, or billing codes, or malpractice insurance. We don't teach them how to recognize a toxic workplace or how to say no to a predatory job offer. We don't teach them how to lead teams, manage staff, or navigate ethical complexity beyond the exam room.

Instead, we focus on compliance. On multiple-choice tests. On systems that reward regurgitation over reflection. And in doing so, we leave our students exquisitely trained for the clinical exam—and utterly unprepared for the professional realities that follow.

Equally concerning is the pervasive failure of the medical education system to recognize and support the personal ambition and individual calling of each physician. Medical education scholars and policymakers tend to treat physicians as if they were uniformly capable of overcoming all professional obstacles without any differentiated support. This is a damaging illusion.

I remember what it felt like to enter practice with that kind of blind spot. When I finished residency, I felt ready for anything inside the hospital. But I was completely unprepared for everything outside it. I didn't understand how billing worked. I didn't know how to evaluate a contract. I didn't even know what questions to ask during negotiations. I assumed good clinical work would be enough. It wasn't.

What followed for me (and for too many others) was a series of hard lessons.

You cannot keep sending students into practice unarmed. If they leave your classrooms without understanding contracts, billing systems, negotiation, or the business of medicine, then we have failed them. They need financial literacy, practice management, and entrepreneurial thinking just as much as they need pathology and physiology. These are not extras; they are survival skills. If you teach them, students will enter the profession with clarity and confidence instead of confusion and fear.

These lessons came not in lecture halls, but in lawyers' offices, courtroom hearings, and moments of private despair. No one ever told me how easily your career can be undone by things that have nothing to do with clinical skill. I had to learn the rules the hard way. And by the time I did, the damage had already been done.

There is little to no infrastructure in place to help physicians who may not be the most assertive or business-savvy to succeed and grow. These physicians are left to struggle in silence, often judged as failures rather than being supported with tools to elevate their performance, income, and career fulfillment.

Medical education must evolve, not by abandoning scientific rigor but by expanding the definition of what it means to be a physician. Future MDs need more than facts. They need context. They need tools to lead. They need preparation not only for boards but also for boardrooms.

Imagine a curriculum that includes negotiation training. Leadership development. Conflict resolution. Ethics in systems design. Financial literacy. Legal literacy. Emotional resilience. Imagine a hidden curriculum that is no longer hidden, where the unspoken lessons are made explicit, examined, and improved.

Imagine if we stopped pretending that burnout is a personal failure and started teaching students how to spot systemic dysfunction. Imagine if we taught them how to speak up—safely, strategically, and with support.

Medical education and professional development programs must evolve to support the individual ambitions and callings of physicians. Personalized mentoring, flexible training tracks, and career path innovation must be part of every stage of a physician's development.

The students you are training today will inherit a healthcare system in flux. They will face challenges your generation never imagined. But they also carry the potential to reimagine what medicine becomes next.

Give them the tools to do that.

Don't just teach them how to pass exams. Teach them how to survive systems. Teach them how to lead with clarity, humility, and courage.

Because what they don't learn in your classrooms, they will have to learn in courtrooms. In crisis. In moments of costly silence.

You are not just educators. You are architects of the future. And the foundation you lay will determine how well the next generation of physicians can navigate a system in flux. By expanding what we teach to include leadership, business acumen, ethics, and resilience, we equip students not just to survive but also to shape what comes next. Let us meet this moment with foresight and courage, knowing that the changes we make now will ripple forward through every life they touch.

CHAPTER 18

To Medical Students and Residents: Stay Human, Stay Awake

You came to this profession with hope. You brought intellect, discipline, and sacrifice. You came with an ache to help, to heal, to matter.

And yet, you may already feel disillusioned.

You are not imagining it. The culture of medicine is deeply flawed.

You are entering a system that demands a great deal and offers little clarity in return. You are told to be compassionate while being trained in environments that reward detachment. You are told to be team players while being isolated by schedules, exams, and unspoken hierarchies. You are asked to make decisions with moral weight, without the safety of mentorship or the space to reflect.

You have likely seen how medicine idealizes self-sacrifice. You may have internalized the belief that needing rest is a sign of weakness. That setting boundaries is selfish. That questioning authority is unprofessional. But none of that is true. These are remnants of a broken system that has passed down its dysfunction as tradition.

I remember how early the erosion began. During residency, I learned how to disassociate from myself: to ignore my body's signals, suppress my emotions, and keep moving forward through anything. I thought that was a strength. But all I was doing was practicing how to disappear. I kept trying to mold myself into a shape that would fit a system built on silence and survival. Eventually, I realized that wasn't sustainable.

What I wish someone had told me is what I am telling you now: Your humanity is not a liability. It is your anchor. Your greatest asset. And if you want a career that lasts, you must protect it. You must protect yourself.

Learn to listen when something feels wrong. That feeling is data. Learn to speak up when boundaries are crossed. Silence will not save you. Learn to rest, not as a reward, but as a requirement. Learn that your worth is not in how many hours you work but in the clarity and compassion you bring to your work.

You are not weak. You are awake.

And we need you to stay awake because your awareness is part of what will change this profession.

You deserve mentors who are honest about the challenges ahead. You deserve training environments that teach emotional resilience, not just clinical knowledge. You deserve transparency about career paths, compensation, and contract negotiations. You deserve to be treated not as a future cog in a machine but as a future colleague and leader.

If something feels off, say so. If a practice model seems unethical, ask why. If a teaching moment crosses a line, name it. More people than you think will stand with you, but they need to see someone go first.

You don't have to burn out to belong. You don't have to become cynical to survive. You can ask for help. You can demand change. You can choose a path that reflects your values, even if it means walking away from traditional routes.

I didn't leave medicine because I lacked skill. I left because I couldn't keep practicing in a system that punished integrity and ignored pain. I share my story not to scare you, but to prepare you. To give you an idea of what you can expect. To remind you that you are not alone.

There is another way to practice. But you will have to fight for it. You will have to build it, often while still managing to survive the current one. And that is hard. But it is worth it.

Because the world still needs physicians like you, not just for your brains, but for your hearts. Not just for your training, but for your conscience.

This profession is worth fighting for. But it's only worth it if you can do it without losing yourself.

So stay curious. Stay honest. Stay human.

Medicine needs you, not as a replica of what has been, but as an architect of what could be.

These problems are complex, but the first steps do not have to be. Here are actions that physicians, schools, and advocacy groups can take right now.

For independent practices and physician groups:

- Build a payer command center with denial heatmaps and monthly scorecards.
- Launch a ten-measure dashboard and suspend all other metrics for 90 days.
- Add scribe or voice tools in the most burdened specialties.
- Create a negotiation playbook that bans retro denials and sets appeal timelines.
- Join or form a consortium to share analytics and negotiating leverage.

For medical schools and residencies:

- Adopt the medical business curriculum and require a capstone.
- Add a clinician-executive certificate that can roll into a future degree.

For state societies and advocacy groups:

- Push for a Physician Due Process Act.
- Back prior authorization reform, including gold-carding and fast tracks.
- Demand specialty-matched peer review and published board decisions.

Real reform will take time, but progress begins when someone takes the first step. If we wait for permission, nothing will change. If we act, even in small ways, the system will begin to shift.

CHAPTER 19

To Insurance Companies

If there is one place where every physician, regardless of specialty, feels the weight of a system pressing against them, it is in the maze of prior authorizations.

These battles do not make care safer. They do not make care better. They make care slower, harder, and, for too many patients, unavailable when it matters most. And they have become so routine that we almost forget how much damage they do.

To reclaim medicine, we have to name what corrupted it. And that means naming the Medical Deep State: the networks of influence that have turned care into compliance and healing into hierarchy.

For decades now, doctors have been told to simply "work through the process." But the process is not neutral. It is a barrier, and every barrier has a cost.

Here is what that cost looks like when you are the one trying to care for someone in need:

1. **Denials that defy medical judgment**
   Procedures, lab tests, and surgeries are denied on the basis of internal guidelines that have little to do with clinical

standards. Doctors appeal—sometimes more than once—while patients wait, conditions worsen, and emergencies become inevitable.

2. **Dangerous delays**
   Even when care is eventually approved, those approvals often take days or weeks. That time is not harmless. It narrows the treatment window. It fuels anxiety. It erodes trust. Patients blame their doctors, not knowing that the delay is coming from somewhere else entirely.

3. **Disrupted schedules, disrupted lives**
   When approval finally comes, hospitals and surgical centers scramble to rework schedules. Operating rooms are double-booked. Patients are asked to rearrange their lives with only a few days' notice. Staff are burned out from the constant reshuffling.

4. **Opaque rules, no clear reasons**
   Denials often arrive without any explanation and without any criteria to meet next time. Phone calls yield little more than scripted answers. Physicians are left guessing at invisible standards.

5. **Decisions made by people who are not clinicians**
   Many prior authorization reviews are conducted by clerical or non-clinical staff who work from lists instead of judgment. These rejections should never have been made, yet physicians must spend valuable time proving what should have been obvious from the start.

6. **An administrative burden that strangles care**
   Many hours each week, often 12 or more, are consumed by paperwork, phone calls, and appeals. This time does not heal a single patient. It only pushes doctors closer to burnout.

7. **Guidelines frozen in the past**
   Insurance policies often demand outdated steps before granting approval—like months of conservative treatment for injuries that modern medicine knows require immediate repair. These rules ignore evidence. They prolong suffering.

8. **Undermining evidence-based care**
   Physicians are second-guessed by cost-driven algorithms. Evidence is pushed aside. Patients watch their doctor's recommendations being overruled by a company they've never met.

9. **Repeat authorizations for chronic conditions**
   Even when a diagnosis is clear and ongoing, every lab, every scan, every procedure must be authorized again. The cycle repeats endlessly.

10. **Financial harm and emotional toll**
    When care is denied or delayed, some patients pay out of pocket. Many cannot. They live with pain and with fear, wondering why a system designed to help them seems determined to block them.

These are not inconveniences. They are harms. And when physicians speak about the causes of exhaustion of modern medicine, prior authorization is almost always near the top of the list.

In June 2025, during a roundtable meeting—brought together by Dr. Mehmet Oz and Robert F. Kennedy Jr. (RFK Jr.)—54 insurance executives were asked to commit to reform. Physicians who attended were skeptical. Prior efforts to streamline this process have ended with promises that never became reality.

The truth is that prior authorization, as it exists today, is not a safeguard. It is a wall. And every day that wall stands, physicians are forced to climb it while patients wait on the other side.

This is not sustainable. If insurance companies do not lead the change, physicians will be forced to. Because we know what is at stake. Behind every form, every delay, every denial, there is a human being who deserves better than a system of obstacles.

CHAPTER 20

To Journalists and Media: Tell the Whole Story

You shape how the public sees medicine. That is not an overstatement. The headlines you write, the stories you chase, the questions you ask define the boundaries of what people seem to understand about healthcare. In moments of crisis, you are often the only translator between the medical world and the rest of the world.

But far too often, the story gets flattened.

Physician burnout is reduced to buzzwords. Complex systemic issues are portrayed as personal failures. The physicians who leave are seen as weak, entitled, or unwilling to adapt. And the ones who stay are rarely asked how they're managing to endure.

In the public eye, physicians are still portrayed as elite and overpaid, immune to economic or emotional hardship. That framing is not just outdated; it's dangerous. It obscures the real story: The medical profession is hemorrhaging its most committed people, not because they no longer care, but because they have been pushed to the edge by systems that do not care for them.

We don't need more stories that ask, "Why are physicians so burned out?" We need stories that ask, "Who benefits from their burnout?" We don't need another feature on "resilience training."

We need an investigation into why healthcare employers continue to prescribe it instead of addressing the underlying issues.

There are stories waiting to be told. Stories like the physician who quit after a hospital merger turned her team into a spreadsheet. The rural practice closed because its electronic records system made it impossible to bill accurately. The resident who looked up one day and realized that every attending she admired had either retired early or switched careers.

If you want to serve the public, tell the whole story. Tell the stories of harm, but also the stories of resistance. Tell what's happening inside statehouses, boardrooms, residency lounges, and consulting firms. Ask why we keep trying to fix medicine without listening to the people who actually deliver care.

The best journalism doesn't just report facts; it reveals patterns. It connects dots that people don't yet know need connecting. And in this moment, perhaps no story is more important than the quiet exodus of physicians who believed medicine was a calling, only to find themselves caught in a system that does not value the very things they were taught to uphold.

We need your voice. Your curiosity. Your ability to question what others accept as normal. Tell the story behind the story because medicine, and the people it serves, are depending on it.

CHAPTER 21

To Employers, Recruiters, and Contract Negotiators: Stop Exploiting the Naive

You are often the first point of contact for a physician stepping into the workforce. You hold the pen that writes the terms. You shape the offers that set the tone for entire careers.

And too often, those offers are built not on transparency but on advantage.

Medicine is the only profession in which someone can train for over a decade, accrue hundreds of thousands in debt, and still enter the job market without basic knowledge of how to evaluate a contract. Physicians are experts in science, not business. We've been taught to defer, to comply, to trust.

That makes us vulnerable.

We are vulnerable to contracts with hidden clauses and misunderstood wording. Productivity metrics we don't understand. Non-competes that destroy future options. Compensation packages that reward speed over judgment. Promises made verbally that never appear in writing.

I recall the first contract I signed after completing my residency. I was so excited to have a job. I didn't know what I didn't know. I didn't have a lawyer look at it. I didn't question the structure. I just signed. And it wasn't until I was working 60-hour weeks with no support and no leverage that I realized what I had agreed to.

I speak now not with bitterness, but with clarity. Because what happened to me has happened to far too many others. And it keeps happening because no one is holding the employers accountable.

If you are in a position to hire physicians, you hold immense power. That power can be used to exploit. Or it can be used to steward.

Do not mistake the lack of negotiation as comfort. Physicians may not push back because they don't know how, or because they've been conditioned not to. That doesn't make the contract fair. It makes it dangerous.

When writing offers, ask yourself: Would I sign this if I were in their position? Would I want my own child to accept this deal? Would I feel proud defending this structure in public?

Fairness is not a favor. It is a baseline. And if we want a medical profession that retains talent, we must stop baiting new physicians with promises and trapping them with fine print.

Transparency should be standard. Salary structures should be explainable. Expectations should be clear. The workload should be sustainable. And every offer should come with an invitation to review, reflect, and ask questions without fear.

I still carry the weight of that first contract. It taught me a lot, but at a cost. I had to leave a position I once loved because the terms were stacked against me. I didn't even know I could walk away until it was too late.

Let's stop setting physicians up for that kind of regret.

You can build trust, not just transactions. You can recruit for longevity, not just productivity. You can be part of the solution.

Because when physicians feel respected at the start, they are more likely to stay. To lead. To thrive.

And when they don't, we all lose.

Write better contracts. Offer better terms. Build better relationships.

It's not just good ethics. It's good business.

CHAPTER 22

To Private Practice Physicians: Your Autonomy Still Matters

There was a time when private practice was the heartbeat of American medicine. It was the model that trained us, inspired us, and for many, launched careers defined by service, innovation, and independence. It was not easy. It was never simple. But it was ours.

Today, that model is vanishing. The forces of consolidation, regulation, and corporatization have made private practice feel not just difficult, but almost impossible. Across the country, physicians are selling their practices, not because they want to, but because they feel they have no choice. They are overwhelmed by overhead, bogged down in bureaucracy, and outmatched by health systems with deeper pockets and larger networks.

But even as the numbers shrink, something stubborn remains. A group of physicians—often quiet, often tired, but deeply committed—still believe in the value of independence. They still believe that care can be personal. That medicine is not just a job but a relationship. That autonomy is not a luxury but a responsibility.

To those physicians, this chapter is for you.

You do not need to be told what the fight looks like. You live it. You know what it's like to chase unpaid claims, to navigate changing payer contracts, to fight for fair reimbursement while still showing up at 2 a.m. when a patient needs you. You know what it costs to stay independent. You've paid it in time, in margin, in sleep.

But you also know what it gives back. You know the value of walking into your own exam room, of making decisions based on your patient's needs rather than institutional targets. You know what it means to treat a whole family, to see someone not just as a chart but as a human being you've known for years. That continuity, that trust, is not measurable in RVUs. But it matters. More than ever.

The story we're told is that private practice is outdated. That it's inefficient, disorganized, and incompatible with modern medicine. But that story is written by those who benefit from its disappearance. The truth is that independent physicians often deliver more personalized, cost-effective, and relationship-centered care than their employed counterparts. The problem is not the model. The problem is the system built around it.

That system rewards consolidation. It ties favorable contracts to scale. It drowns small practices in reporting requirements that were designed with hospitals in mind. It imposes technology built for billing departments, not clinicians. And then it blames you for struggling under its weight.

You are not failing. The system is not designed to let you succeed.

But that does not mean you are powerless.

The future of private practice will not look like its past. It will require new thinking, new partnerships, and new protections. It may require joining with other practices to gain leverage or investing in shared infrastructure to reduce costs. It may mean learning more about business than you ever intended, as well as teaching your teams to think like owners, not just employees.

Elimination of Private Medical Practice

Here are some of the serious consequences that will follow the elimination of private medical practice.

Consequence: Collapse of Physician Autonomy

When physicians lose the freedom to make independent clinical decisions, their role shifts from advocate to employee. In private practice, physicians set their own schedules, choose which patients to see, and determine the course of care. Without that autonomy, their ability to tailor care to individual patients erodes. Decisions are instead driven by protocols, productivity targets, and cost-saving directives issued by distant administrators. As a result, physicians find themselves unable to practice the kind of medicine that drew them to the profession in the first place.

Consequence: Decline in Quality of Patient Care

Independent practices are often where patients receive the most personalized and attentive care. Private physicians tend to have smaller patient panels and more flexibility in how they spend their time. When private practices vanish, patients are absorbed into large systems where encounters are shorter, relationships are thinner, and care is fragmented. The emphasis shifts to throughput and compliance with corporate standards, rather than continuity and outcomes.

Consequence: Increased Physician Burnout

The structure of employed medicine places relentless pressure on physicians. Facing productivity metrics, endless charting requirements, and less control over their time, physicians in corporate systems burn out at alarming rates. Independent practice, while challenging, gives physicians the opportunity to set their own boundaries and rediscover meaning in their work. Without that outlet, many leave medicine entirely, deepening workforce shortages.

Consequence: Skyrocketing Healthcare Costs

Contrary to popular belief, physician-owned practices are often the most cost-effective providers of care. They refer more judiciously, manage care proactively, and avoid unnecessary testing and procedures. Large corporate systems, in contrast, are incentivized to maximize billable services and often operate with far higher overhead. Eliminating private practice opens the floodgates to unchecked billing practices that drive healthcare costs even higher.

Consequence: Worsened Access in Rural and Underserved Areas

Private practices are frequently the last remaining lifeline in medically underserved regions. When those practices close, either from acquisition or lack of support, patients in these areas are left without local care. Large systems rarely invest in rural communities unless there is a financial incentive. The result is longer travel times, delayed diagnoses, and worse outcomes for the patients in greatest need.

Consequence: Erosion of Ethical Standards

The integrity of medicine depends on a sacred trust between doctor and patient. In corporate structures, that trust is compromised. Physicians are routinely pressured to prioritize business goals over clinical judgment. Treatment decisions can be influenced by contracts, performance metrics, or institutional priorities, rather than what is best for the individual patient. The elimination of independent practice strips physicians of the moral authority to stand fully on the side of those they serve.

Consequence: Reduction in Innovation and Entrepreneurship

Some of the most creative and responsive care models have emerged from independent practices. Concierge medicine, direct primary care, and integrative models of treatment all found their footing outside of large systems. Private practice physicians have the agility to try new approaches and build care models tailored to their communities. Corporate medicine, by contrast, is inherently risk-averse and slow to change. Eliminating private practice would choke off a vital source of innovation in American healthcare.

Consequence: Loss of a Foundational American Ideal

Independent medical practice represents more than a business model. It reflects a tradition of service, stewardship, and self-determination. These practices are often embedded in their communities and offer a level of accountability that can't be replicated in centralized systems. Their disappearance would mark the end of a profession once defined by purpose, sacrifice, and freedom. What's lost is not just a practice model but a cornerstone of American medicine.

But we cannot give up.

Because when private practice disappears entirely, essential elements go with it. The ability to say, "I believe this is what my patient needs," and to act on that belief. The ability to set your own pace, build your own culture, and lead your team with integrity. The ability to innovate at the ground level, to adjust quickly, to care deeply, and to stay close to the work that drew you here.

If medicine is to be saved, it will not be saved solely by institutions. It will be saved by people who still believe that care belongs closest to the patient. People who are willing to carry more risk in exchange for more responsibility. People who still believe that autonomy and accountability can coexist.

You are one of those people.

You should not have to do this alone. We need policies that level the playing field, technologies designed for small practices, and payment models that do not punish independence. We need lenders who understand medical business models, and associations that support solo and small-group physicians with real advocacy, not just lip service. We need new pathways for younger physicians who want to build their own practices but cannot imagine how.

But until those systems are built, your voice remains essential. Not as a relic of the past, but as a blueprint for what medicine can still be. You are not holding on to something old. You are holding on to something sacred. And you are proving, every day, that it is still possible to lead with integrity, to practice with freedom, and to serve without compromise.

You are not alone. You are not outdated. You are needed.

And your autonomy still matters.

CHAPTER 23

To Technology Leaders: Build with, Not Around, Physicians

You hold the keys to one of the most powerful forces shaping modern medicine. Not legislation. Not reimbursement. Not even education. You build the tools that define how care is delivered. You create the systems that determine how physicians document, communicate, and spend their time. You decide what fits on the screen and what gets buried. What can be clicked quickly, and what cannot.

Your fingerprints are everywhere, even if you never set foot inside a hospital.

At first, the promise was intoxicating. Technology would liberate physicians. Electronic records would eliminate duplication. Portals would increase access. Artificial intelligence would reduce cognitive load. Workflows would be streamlined. Lives would be saved.

But somewhere between the promise and the product, something went wrong.

What physicians experience is not innovation. It is obstruction. It is the daily frustration of clunky interfaces, nonintuitive menus, broken integrations, and documentation requirements that prioritize billing over care. It is watching patients grow silent while a screen steals the physician's attention. It is finishing a full day of appointments only to face three more hours of charting, inboxes, and click-box fatigue.

This is not what you intended. But it is what you created.

And it happened because too many of these systems were built around physicians, not with them. Their voices were missing in the design phase. Their insights were ignored in implementation. Their concerns were dismissed during testing. The result is technology that is elegant on the backend and exasperating on the front lines.

I remember the day a new system went live in my office. The training was brief, the features complex, and the support minimal. The system didn't understand how I worked. It required six clicks when one click would have been sufficient. It buried critical information under layers of navigation. It offered prompts that contradicted clinical reasoning. And it crashed. Often.

It didn't help me care better. It didn't save time. And it most certainly did not serve the patient.

A system that was missing physicians' voices cost billions to build. But the real cost was less visible. It showed up in burnout rates. In staff turnover. In the steady erosion of trust between clinicians and their tools. And in the moments lost with patients whose eyes never quite met mine because I was trying to find the right checkbox.

You have the power to change this.

Physicians are not anti-technology. They are not resisting the future. They are desperate for tools that make sense. Tools that feel like partners, not burdens. Tools that enhance their judgment, support their decisions, and respect their time. They want systems that are intuitive, responsive, and designed for clinical realities, not compliance optics.

But that kind of technology can only be built one way: with them, not without.

Bring them in from the beginning. Not after the wireframes are finished. Not just to sign off on usability testing. But at the table, from day one. Ask them what they need. Watch how they work. Sit with them through a full day and feel what they feel when the system slows down. Listen not just to what they say, but also to what exhausts them, what they avoid, and what they trust.

Then build with that in mind.

Because the goal is not just more technology; it is better medicine. And medicine only gets better when those who practice it are heard, respected, and trusted to shape the tools they use.

This is not just a product problem. It is a power problem. And solving it means recognizing that the people with the most to lose from bad technology are the very people who have been left out of its creation.

If your tool increases the time it takes to document a visit, it is not helping. If it buries clinical nuance in templated language, it is not serving care. If it breaks the patient connection, it is breaking the work itself.

You are in a position to make that change. Not by promising less disruption, but by building with more wisdom. Not by selling another fix, but by slowing down and asking better questions. Not by optimizing for revenue, but by remembering that your product will touch lives you will never meet.

There is a path forward. One where physicians are not just users, but collaborators. Where design reflects reality. Where technology frees clinicians to be more present, more thoughtful, and more human.

Medicine does not need more features. It needs more listening. And your greatest innovation may not be your next release. It may be the moment you finally decide to build with, not around, the people whose hands will carry your work into the lives of others.

They are ready to help. Let them in.

CHAPTER 24

We Do What We Can and Hope for the Best

Physicians did not enter this profession because we wanted to build unions or wage political battles. We came here to heal. Yet over time, we have learned that passion and skill are not enough to protect a career. Medicine is a calling, but it is also a business. And when we are sent into that business without the tools to navigate it, the cost is staggering.

Fifty years ago, there was talk of creating a unified physician voice, but the effort collapsed. The collapse was not because doctors did not care. It was because we struggled to align. Each of us builds a practice in our own way. That independence, while deeply valuable, has also kept us from acting together when it matters most.

This fragmentation has a price. It leaves us exposed to the same forces that have been hollowing out private practice for decades. Government mandates, payer restrictions, corporate control, and a steady erosion of respect have pushed physicians to the edge. Burnout now affects more than 70 percent of us. And many who once felt called to this work now feel they have no choice but to leave it.

The heart of the problem is that medical training has never taught physicians how to run a business. Those who succeed in private practice usually do so not by due diligence, but by stumbling into a specialty with better margins, or by developing leadership skills on their own. For most, the lack of preparation becomes clear only after years of struggle. By then, the damage is often done.

If nothing changes, the trajectory is predictable. Consolidation. Employment. Control of medical decisions by people who have never treated a patient. And as the workforce shifts, an increasing reliance on physicians trained in socialized systems overseas. Many of these doctors are competent and hardworking. But their training models often emphasize volume over relationship. That is not a criticism of them. It is a description of the conditions that shaped them. And it is a warning that our own system is headed in the same direction.

Every year, the machinery grows heavier. More rules. More reporting. More productivity requirements. Fewer choices. We are being turned into parts of a system that no longer trusts us to do the very thing we were trained to do. That is why understanding the business of medicine is no longer optional. It is the difference between being able to build a career on your own terms or being absorbed into a system that decides for you. All choices are lost.

Business knowledge does not mean abandoning medicine. It means protecting it. It gives a physician the power to structure a practice, set a course, and stay independent. It is the only path that allows a doctor to control their own future.

Today, there are a few models that offer a way forward. Direct primary care allows patients to pay a monthly fee for unlimited access without the interference of insurers. Concierge medicine, often for higher-income patients, gives physicians a similar degree of control with a focus on time and relationship. And physician-owned cooperatives or networks allow independent practices to join together for scale and negotiating strength without giving up autonomy.

These approaches are not perfect. They take planning, courage, and the willingness to think differently. They also require us to confront a painful truth: The current medical system is not coming to save us. There are no plans from medical schools, from Congress, or from national organizations that will turn the tide.

If we want change, we will have to build it ourselves.

That is why the idea of physician-owned cooperatives deserves serious attention. When solo practitioners group together under a common business structure, they gain the leverage to negotiate better contracts, share costs, and protect their independence. They can decide how to practice instead of waiting for permission. The larger these groups become, the stronger they get. They will not fix everything. But they are a practical starting point.

The same holds true in rural areas, where options are even more limited. Physicians there face the same pressures as those in cities, only with fewer patients and resources. Many of them will be forced into hospital employment just to survive. That is why the cooperative model is especially critical in places where isolation has left physicians with almost no support.

This is the reality. Unless physicians learn the language of business and stand together, the profession will continue to slide toward a system in which autonomy is gone. The result will be a medical landscape dominated by large entities that dictate how care is delivered, leaving doctors as functionaries in someone else's machine.

There is still time to act. Independent physicians can choose a different path. They can choose to learn what they were never taught. They can choose to join forces instead of struggling alone. And they can choose to practice in ways that protect their ability to care.

I know what it feels like to lose a practice. To walk out of an office for the last time and know that everything you built is gone. I know what it is to take whatever work you can find just to stay connected to medicine. And I know how hard it is to keep believing that the work matters when the system seems determined to grind you down.

But I also know this. Every doctor who still chooses to stay in this fight matters. Every doctor who chooses to learn the business side of medicine, who chooses to build or join a cooperative, who chooses to keep the exam room a place of trust and humanity, makes a difference.

We cannot fix everything overnight. We can do what we can. We can keep going. And we can hope for the best. Because if enough of us make that choice, it may be enough to begin again.

But knowing the solutions is not enough. We must also be honest about what brought us to this point. Burnout is not a failure of character. It is not about grit, or stamina, or the willingness to tough it out. It is the natural result of practicing medicine in a system that has stripped away meaning, autonomy, and trust.

Physicians today are being asked to do more than ever in environments that value speed over skill, efficiency over empathy, and documentation over discernment. They spend their days fighting with insurance companies, managing bureaucratic tasks, and navigating a maze of regulations that make care harder instead of easier. Many spend more time with screens than with patients.

Worse still, the system often blames them for the damage it inflicts. Instead of addressing the root causes, leadership offers surface solutions (wellness modules, mindfulness apps, or scheduled resilience training), acting as if the problem lies with the doctor, not the design.

This is more than exhausting. It is a violation of what the profession was meant to be.

The physicians who leave are not giving up. They are responding to a system that makes it impossible to practice with integrity. What they walk away from is not medicine, but rather the machinery that has made medicine unrecognizable. And what they feel is not relief, but grief.

If we continue to ignore the forces driving this exodus and keep treating burnout as a private problem rather than a systemic one, we will lose doctors. And not only will we lose doctors, but also what made medicine worth practicing.

Now is the time to listen. And more that that. Now is the time to act.

Part 4
Rebuilding Medicine from the Inside Out

CHAPTER 25

Solution: Eliminate Policy Structures That Harm

Many of the policies governing American medicine were created with good intentions. But intentions do not insulate a policy from its consequences. In fact, some of the most well-meaning structures in healthcare are doing the most harm, not because they are malicious, but because they were designed without physicians at the table.

When we pass policy without understanding what physicians actually do, we create systems that look rational on paper but fall apart in practice. We design quality metrics that don't measure quality. We impose billing requirements that don't reflect clinical complexity. We assign value based on codes, not care.

These policies are not just frustrating. They are destructive. They turn physicians into box-checkers. They reward compliance over wisdom. They push MDs into moral distress by forcing them to choose between what is best for their patients and what is required by the system.

Medical doctors in Congress are suppressed. Their voices are dismissed, and they rarely have the power or status to push through medical reforms that matter. Most stay silent and do what is expected of them. When meaningful legislation comes up, such as making malpractice insurance more equitable, the voices of physicians are quickly drowned out. Lobbyists for insurance companies and the attorneys who dominate the legislative ranks press their advantage, and their influence prevails. The legal profession has turned malpractice into a profitable enterprise, and any attempt to provide physicians with greater protection is intentionally blocked. Lawmakers care little about the stress, fear, and financial strain that drive physicians out of medicine.

Even physicians who are also attorneys witness the reality of this imbalance, both in the courtroom and in legislative debate. They see clearly that the money always wins. Doctors have learned that resistance is futile, and many have accepted the culture of "go along to get along." The result is a system in which the expertise of medical professionals is sidelined and the profession itself is weakened by the weight of politics and profit.

We must begin by reviewing existing policies through a new lens: one that centers on physician insight, patient outcomes, and ethical care. That means inviting frontline clinicians into the policy conversation, and not as a token presence, but as essential architects.

It means eliminating requirements that serve no clinical purpose. It means resisting the urge to solve every problem with a new regulation. And it means acknowledging that when physicians leave the profession because of policy-induced burnout, those policies have failed.

We also need guardrails to prevent future harm. Every new policy should undergo a physician impact assessment: a systematic review of how the proposed change will affect the daily work and well-being of healthcare providers. This should not be a rubber stamp. It should be a rigorous and transparent process that elevates physician voices and surfaces unintended consequences before they cause real harm.

Policy can be a force for good, but only if it is shaped by those who understand the realities of care. If we want to build a better system, we must stop mistaking paperwork for progress and start listening to the people on whom medicine depends.

CHAPTER 26

Solution: Enforce Ethical Standards in Health Management

A system is only as ethical as the people empowered to run it. For decades, healthcare institutions have been led by individuals trained in business rather than medicine. Some have done so honorably. Others have prioritized profits, metrics, and market dominance over the well-being of patients and physicians.

This happened to me while serving in a hospital in Michigan, and it is not an understatement to say that the problems it caused were manifold. The first problem arose when it came to assigning leadership. I had multiple years of experience in OB/GYN and was the logical person to appoint to head up a team of nine nurse practitioner midwives who helped with pregnancies, labors, and deliveries. Instead of giving that role to me, the administrator chose a millionaire doctor with political influence in the community. He neglected to give me the leadership, even though I was much more experienced.

This resulted in a situation where an unnecessary C-section took place. The protocol at the hospital was that when one of the midwives had a problem, they would call the doctor on duty, who would come up and give advice and intercede where required.

I received one such call. It was from a panicked midwife who was sure a baby she was delivering was going to die. She was basing her opinion on the fetal scalp monitor attached to the baby's head as it was progressing in labor. I complied with her request, examined the history of the fetal strip, and concluded that the baby was fine. There was nothing to be overly concerned about.

Instead of accepting my experienced, professional diagnosis, she called in a different doctor. He immediately performed a C-section. Not because it was in the mother's and child's best interest, but because it was the easy decision to make and hide behind.

When I saw him later and asked him about the situation, he apologized. He acknowledged that the strip was normal, but if you looked at it over a long period of time, he saw "a bit of a dip." He said that had been a part of his training. Thankfully, the mother and child both ended up healthy. But an unnecessary C-section was performed.

That hospital in Michigan had around ten OBG staff members. I had over eight years of experience using an ultrasound in my office, whereas none of the staff there had any experience. I also had ten years of experience doing laparoscopic procedures before joining this hospital staff. None of the OBG staff were proficient in laparoscopic surgery. The hospital and staff were eight years behind in these skills, and the CEO made no effort to let me teach them how to use these tools, even when I offered.

In another instance, the CEO refused to let his team be trained in cutting-edge technology. I had the background and experience that would have served the hospital and patients well. It had to do with laparoscopic surgery. It allowed us to do tubal ligations more effectively and with much less risk to the patient.

I was told that they had all of the equipment needed to implement this new technique. A test case was scheduled for me to demonstrate the new procedure. When I arrived in the operating room, the nurse opened the laparoscopic instruments tray. To my surprise, most of the routine laparoscopic instruments used in most procedures were missing and had never been ordered! I was only able to partially complete the procedure.

Then, when I was performing another procedure, there was an issue with the trocar, which is a very wide piece of straight metal that is narrowed down to a small point and used to make a hole in the abdomen. The instrument was so dull that it brought into play the possibility of accidentally cutting the patient's aorta. I immediately ended the surgery.

Instead of thanking me for pointing out these shortcomings, I was reported to the surgery committee with the accusation of incompetence. These types of occurrences are not rare; in fact, they happen on a regular basis. Personal emotion and political considerations trump what is best for the patients in our care.

We cannot afford to look away. As long as healthcare leaders can act without accountability to the people whom their decisions most affect, the profession and its patients will suffer.

Codes of ethics bind physicians, and those who manage them should have similar codes. Health system executives, insurance administrators, and other non-clinical decision-makers wield tremendous power over clinical outcomes. Yet there is no binding ethical standard to guide their actions, nor is there meaningful oversight to assess the real-world effects of their decisions.

This is not simply a governance issue. It is a moral crisis. When hospital administrators reduce staffing to cut costs, knowing it will compromise care, they are making a choice with significant ethical implications. When insurance companies deny coverage for necessary treatment based on opaque algorithms, they are not just managing risk; they are practicing medicine without responsibility.

The same thing happens when a radiologist reads the film of a patient and fails to see breast cancer present. Who gets sued? The surgeon who accepted the diagnosis of no cancer until it spread and it was too late to save a life.

It is time to change that. Healthcare administrators should be held to a formal, transparent code of ethics that prioritizes patient care, clinician well-being, and integrity over financial considerations. Their decisions should be subject to review by ethical boards composed of physicians. And their compensation should be tied not only to financial outcomes but also to clinical and ethical ones.

Medical boards hold physicians accountable. We need structures that do the same for healthcare leaders. Until we do, we will continue to see physicians punished for moral decisions that administrators make easy to ignore.

Ethics cannot be optional in healthcare leadership. They must be embedded in every level of decision-making, from boardrooms to budget meetings. Because in a system where business often trumps care, we must have the courage to demand better from those who shape the rules.

CHAPTER 27

Solution: Physician-Centered Technology

Technology in healthcare promised to make everything easier: More accurate records, better communication, and faster care. Instead, it has become one of the most cited sources of physician frustration. Electronic health records are cumbersome. Documentation requirements are excessive. The time spent on screens now routinely exceeds the time spent with patients.

This is not a failure of innovation. It is a failure of design.

Most healthcare technology is not designed with physicians in mind. It is built for billing departments, compliance officers, and data analysts. The user experience for clinicians is often an afterthought, if considered at all. The result is technology that obstructs rather than supports the delivery of care.

To reverse this trend, we must radically reorient our approach. Technology should be developed with physician input from day one. That means involving physicians not only in usability testing but in initial planning, prototyping, and decision-making. If a tool does not improve clinical care or reduce cognitive load, it does not belong in the physician's workflow.

We need systems that are intuitive, responsive, and customizable to different specialties. We need decision-support tools that enhance clinical judgment instead of undermining it. We also need to measure success not just by the data captured but also by the time restored to physicians and patients.

The goal is not to eliminate technology. It is to serve those who serve others. When technology respects the physician's time, attention, and expertise, it becomes what it was always meant to be: a partner in care.

If we want to retain our best physicians, we must stop designing tools that treat them like data-entry clerks. We must build systems that reflect the realities of clinical life and the humanity of those who practice it. Physician-centered technology is not a luxury. It is a necessity.

CHAPTER 28

Solution: A National Campaign for Physician Respect

The cultural story we tell about physicians has drifted. Once seen as trusted leaders and advocates for the public good, many physicians now feel reduced to service providers, cost centers, or obstacles in a system designed by others. This shift is not just unfortunate; it is corrosive.

Respect is not a perk. It is the foundation of professional sustainability. When physicians are consistently spoken of in transactional or adversarial terms, it undermines their morale, their credibility, and their willingness to stay in a profession that demands so much.

We need a new story.

We need a national campaign: not a PR initiative, but a collective cultural reckoning with the truth of what physicians actually do and why it matters. This campaign should highlight the value of the medical profession to society, celebrate physicians who model integrity and courage, and tell the real stories behind the headlines.

It should be led by physicians but supported by institutions, media, educators, and patients. It should appear in classrooms, newsrooms, boardrooms, and political conversations. And it should be grounded in truth—not flattery, not nostalgia, but an honest recognition of how deeply medicine has shaped the lives of every person in this country.

Rebuilding respect does not mean shielding physicians from accountability. It means refusing to treat them as if they are disposable. It means remembering that care depends not just on clinical skill, but also on the moral and emotional presence of the person offering it. And it means stating, loudly and publicly, that we cannot afford to lose those people.

If we want to keep our physicians, we must restore respect for what they represent. Not just in healthcare. But in the medical culture at large.

CHAPTER 29

Solution: Compensation Models That Align with Purpose

Every profession tells its members what it values, not just through words, but also through what it rewards. In medicine, we emphasize the importance of valuing clinical judgment, compassion, excellence, and service. But the way we compensate physicians often tells a very different story.

In most health systems, a physician's worth is measured in Relative Value Units, productivity targets, and throughput. Time spent thinking, teaching, collaborating, or simply listening is rarely taken into account. The incentive structure is designed for volume, not value. For many, that creates a quiet but corrosive tension between what they believe their work is for and what the system seems to want from them.

I remember the first time I felt it. I had just come from a long consultation with a patient who had suffered multiple pregnancy losses. She was anxious, grieving, and unsure whether to try again. We talked for nearly an hour. I walked her through her options, answered her questions, and gave her the space to feel what she was feeling. It was one of those encounters that reminded me why I became a physician in the first place.

Later that day, I was pulled aside by an administrator. My patient numbers were slipping. I wasn't meeting my targets. The message was clear: Spending time like that, while meaningful, was inefficient.

That moment lodged itself in my chest. It wasn't the first time I had gone "over schedule," and it wouldn't be the last. But it was one of the first times I realized how completely divorced the compensation model was from the actual practice of medicine as I understood it. I wasn't being paid to care. I was being paid to move.

This is not just a management problem. It is a moral one. When the compensation structure rewards speed over thought, volume over nuance, and compliance over character, we begin to lose what medicine is meant to be. We send quiet messages to our physicians: Don't slow down. Don't go deep. Don't take the time you know your patients need. Just keep moving.

Over time, those messages accumulate. Physicians who once took pride in their thoughtfulness begin to cut corners, not out of laziness or indifference but out of self-preservation. They see colleagues rewarded for doing less well, but doing it faster. They see systems that pretend to measure quality but actually measure output. And they feel the slow erosion of purpose.

Compensation is never neutral. It teaches. It shapes. It creates pressure in some places and silence in others. If we want physicians to practice with integrity, presence, and care, then we must stop penalizing those behaviors financially.

That means asking difficult questions. What would it look like to reward complexity rather than volume? How do we value the physician who takes extra time to explain, teach, and advocate? How do we recognize the work that doesn't fit neatly into billing codes but is essential to good care? For example, the hours that physicians remain on the labor and delivery floor during a patient's progress are never paid for.

These are not theoretical concerns. They are questions of design. And design is changeable.

Some systems have begun experimenting with hybrid models that incorporate salary stability, quality metrics based on patient outcomes, and incentives for leadership, teaching, and teamwork. Others are exploring capitation models with accountability for both cost and care. Still others are shifting decision-making power back to physicians themselves, trusting them to define what good looks like and how it should be measured.

None of these models are perfect. But they all start from a different premise: that if you want physicians to stay in the profession, you must pay them in a way that honors why they came to it.

When I think back on the moments that mattered most in my career, none of them show up in my productivity reports. They live in quiet rooms, in hard conversations, and in long hours spent with patients who needed more than the system allowed. I never got a bonus for those moments. But I carry them with me still, because they reminded me of who I was trying to be.

I was never compensated for the countless hours I spent on the labor and delivery floors, consulting with mothers and checking on their progress. No, there was only a certain number of hours I was allowed to bill for, regardless of the additional care I provided. This system de-incentivizes the care that every patient deserves.

We need a system that remembers those moments. Not because they are profitable, but because they are the soul of the work. Compensation models will never capture everything. However, they can do better than they are currently doing. They can reflect not just what we can measure, but what we value.

And if we want physicians to keep giving their best, we must stop asking them to choose between what is right and what is rewarded.

We must give them both.

CHAPTER 30

Solution: Restore Clinical Autonomy

A formal education will make you a living.
Self-education will make you a fortune.

—Jim Rohn

There was a time when physicians were trusted to make decisions. Not perfect decisions, not unchecked or infallible ones, but decisions grounded in years of training, proximity to the patient, and a deep sense of responsibility. That trust—the space to think, to discern, to act—was what made the work not only possible but also meaningful.

Now, for many physicians, that space has disappeared.

Today's physicians work under a kind of quiet surveillance. Their clinical judgment is often second-guessed by algorithms, administrators, and rigid protocols designed without regard for complexity. They are told what tests to order, what medications to prescribe, how many minutes to spend, and how many boxes to check. They are given tools that pretend to support but actually constrain, systems that reduce medicine to a script.

And when they deviate from the script, even for good reason, they are often punished—not explicitly, but through reprimands, poor evaluations, denied authorizations, and subtle warnings that remind them of their place.

I remember the first time I truly felt that loss. I had a patient with an uncommon presentation, something that didn't fit the textbook but that I recognized from experience. I made a clinical decision based on the full picture, including history, labs, behavior, and a dozen other things that don't show up on a spreadsheet. It was the right call. The patient improved.

But later, during a case review, I was questioned for deviating from protocol. The guideline didn't apply to this case, not really, but that didn't matter. The reviewer wasn't in the room. They didn't know the patient. They just knew I hadn't followed the flowchart. That was enough to flag the encounter as problematic.

I wasn't disciplined. But I wasn't supported either. And the message was clear: Stick to the script, even when it makes no sense.

This is the quiet erosion that physicians face. Not overt censorship, but a thousand small constraints that, over time, reshape the very nature of the work. Clinical autonomy becomes the exception, not the rule. Judgment becomes risky. Creativity is discouraged. And the practice of medicine begins to feel like compliance management rather than patient care.

Some say this is necessary. That autonomy must be limited to ensure safety, consistency, and accountability. But that argument assumes a binary: total freedom or total control. What physicians are asking for is something different. They are asking for shared trust. For the freedom to apply their expertise within systems that understand what expertise is. They are asking not to be unaccountable, but to be heard.

Restoring clinical autonomy does not mean abandoning standards. It means recognizing that standards are most powerful when they are guided by wisdom, not enforced by fear. It means creating environments in which physicians can speak up, slow down, and make decisions that reflect the full reality of the person in front of them.

It also means shifting the power dynamic. Too many decisions that affect patient care are made far from the bedside. Formularies are set by insurance companies. Staffing models are decided by finance teams. Protocols are written by committees that rarely include the physicians expected to follow them. The people who know the most about the work often have the least say in how it is structured.

If we want medicine to be thoughtful, we must trust the thinkers. That means building clinical leadership into every level of decision-making. It means letting physicians lead not just in theory but also in practice. It means asking them what they need and then acting on their responses.

Autonomy is not just about control. It is about dignity. It's about knowing that your voice matters, that your training is respected, and that your presence in the room is not just tolerated but essential.

When physicians have autonomy, they stay longer. They give more. They teach, lead, and innovate. They take risks when it matters and hold the line when it counts. But when autonomy is stripped away, something deeper is lost. Not just motivation, but identity.

I did not become a physician to follow orders. I became an MD to care, listen, and make judgments that could change a life. Most physicians I know share the same sentiment. They are not asking for perfection. They are asking for the freedom to bring their full selves to work.

We cannot restore that with slogans. We can only restore it by returning authority to those who carry the weight of responsibility. By honoring clinical judgment. By listening before we regulate. By remembering that systems do not deliver the best care; rather, it is delivered by people with the courage and freedom to do what is right. As Dr. Oz says, "If you mix politics with medicine, you only get politics."

Autonomy is not a luxury. It is a precondition for good medicine. And if we want our physicians to stay, to lead, and to thrive, we must begin by giving them back what the system has quietly taken away.

We must give them room to think. Room to care. Room to decide.

CHAPTER 31

Solution: Business Literacy in Medical Training

There are things every physician remembers about their training. The first patient they lost. The first night on call. The overwhelming volume of information. The pride of surviving it. The fear of getting it wrong.

What most don't remember is a single hour spent learning how the business of medicine actually works—and for a simple reason. No such time exists.

Not how to profit. Not how to climb a corporate ladder. Just the basics. How money moves through a practice. How hospitals set compensation. How insurance companies reimburse. How to read a contract, evaluate a job offer, or decide whether a partnership is fair.

Medical schools do not teach these things. And then we act surprised when physicians are confused, exploited, or burned out. We send them into a complex, high-stakes industry without showing them how that industry functions. We call medicine a profession, but we train our professionals as if they will be shielded from everything outside the exam room.

They will not be.

From the first job interview to the last day of practice, physicians are required to navigate systems shaped by money, management, and metrics. They are asked to negotiate salaries, evaluate productivity models, manage staff, and operate within frameworks they never learned to interpret. And when things go wrong, when they find themselves in contracts that don't protect them or in systems that punish good care, they blame themselves. They assume they missed something. And in a way, they did. But not because they were careless. Because they were never taught.

I know this pattern because I lived it. I remember signing my first employment contract and skipping over the parts I didn't understand. I assumed they were standard. I assumed someone would explain them. No one did. Years later, when the terms of that contract were used against me, I realized how vulnerable I had been. Not because I lacked intelligence, but because I lacked language. I couldn't speak the language of the system I was in.

That is what business literacy is. It is language. And language is power.

When physicians don't know how to discuss revenue, overhead, or reimbursement structures, they are excluded from conversations that directly affect their work. When they don't understand balance sheets or budgets, they can't advocate effectively for resources. When they don't know how compensation is calculated, they can't tell when it's unfair.

That ignorance is not accidental. It is inherited. It is built into a training culture that romanticizes self-sacrifice and distrusts anything that appears to be business-driven. For generations, we've been told that physicians should stay focused on patients, that talking about money is beneath the profession. But while we've stayed silent, others have filled the gap. Administrators. Consultants. Middlemen. People who may or may not understand the realities of care, but who know how to run a meeting, write a contract, and protect their own interests and incomes.

Physicians deserve that same fluency. Not to replace their clinical knowledge, but to strengthen it. To defend it. To lead with it.

Business education should not be delayed until ten years into a career. It should begin during medical school. It should be part of the curriculum, not an elective. It should be taught with the same seriousness we bring to anatomy or pharmacology because understanding how systems work is not a distraction from care. It is part of care.

Students should graduate not only knowing how to diagnose a disease, but also how to evaluate an employment offer. Not only how to write an order, but also how to read a profit and loss statement. Not only how to survive training, but also how to build a sustainable medical practice business, which is the source of their potential success and medical career.

Some schools are starting to make changes for physicians already in practice. They are introducing courses in leadership, finance, negotiation, and health policy. But they don't deal with business marketing and management. The hidden curriculum still teaches that business is someone else's job. That physicians who ask questions about money are less noble. That caring well and managing well are separate things.

They are not.

In my own journey, I learned most of what I know about the business of medicine through personal experience with pain and at my own cost through self-education with a world-renowned business expert, Dan Kennedy. Through mistakes. Through being left out of rooms I didn't even know existed. I don't want that for the next generation. They deserve better. They deserve an education that prepares them not only to care for patients but also to care for their own careers.

Because when physicians are empowered, everything gets better. Decisions are smarter. Teams are stronger. Systems are fairer. Patients receive care that is not only clinically excellent but also structurally supported.

This is not about turning physicians into executives. It is about giving them back their autonomy and freedom to make their own decisions. It is about teaching them the language of power, so they can use it to protect what matters.

No physician should have to learn how the system works only after it harms them. No student should leave training fluent in biochemistry but still struggling with contract negotiations. No profession can thrive if its members don't understand the structures that govern their lives.

It is time to stop pretending that business is outside of a physician's work. It is inside it. And if we want our physicians to lead, to stay, to thrive, we must teach them what the system won't: a business education.

We must teach them how to speak for themselves.

CONCLUSION

We Still Have Time

Medicine is not broken. It is breaking. And that difference matters.

Broken things are abandoned. But things in the process of breaking can still be saved. They can be held together long enough to be reimagined. They can be reinforced, rebuilt, and renewed. They can become stronger, not in spite of their damage, but because we chose not to walk away.

That is the choice before us now.

Across this country, physicians are holding the line. Quietly. Relentlessly. Sometimes at great personal cost. They are staying longer than they should. Carrying more than they can. Working in systems that do not reflect the values that drew them to the profession in the first place.

They are not asking for applause. They are asking for honesty. They are asking for allies. They are asking for a future in which their labor, their judgment, and their presence are no longer treated as expendable.

If that future is going to exist, it will not come from one reform, one election, or one organization. It will come from a thousand conversations, decisions, and refusals. It will come from medical students who ask harder questions, administrators who choose a different metric, and lawmakers who stop listening only to lobbyists. It will come from patients who speak up, reporters who tell the whole story, and physicians who are brave enough to stay in the room and tell the truth.

This book has not offered one single solution. It has offered many. Some will be easy to implement. Others will take years. However, none of these matter if we do not first decide that physicians are worth protecting. That their voices are worth elevating. That the systems they work in should reflect the wisdom they carry.

The work ahead will be uncomfortable. Power rarely shifts without resistance. But that discomfort is a sign that something real is happening. That we are moving from rhetoric to reckoning. That we are no longer content to admire the problem or to mourn what medicine once was. That we no longer have the tolerance we once needed to muster in order to stay in practice.

This is not nostalgia. This is a call to memory. To remember why the profession matters. To remember what care looks like when it is rooted in trust. To remember that the most sacred spaces in medicine are not conference rooms or data dashboards, but the moments between two people, when one is suffering and the other stays.

We still have time to save those moments. But not by waiting. Not by hoping the system corrects itself. We must act.

The question is not whether change is possible. The question is whether we are willing to fight for it.

Because if we are, there is still a future where physicians can thrive. Where their training is honored, their ethics are protected. Where their judgment is trusted. And where their work is shaped not by compliance but by compassion.

That future is not guaranteed. But it is still within reach.

And it begins now.

EPILOGUE

What Nearly Broke Me: And What I Found on the Other Side

From the time I was raised on my grandparents' farm, I learned that strength was quiet, persistent, and earned. My mother, tired of the abuse she endured from my alcoholic father, had brought me to the farm for safety. It was my grandfather—a schoolteacher who had turned to farming—who became my guide.

Cavett Robert once said, "Everybody's walking around with the umbilical cord looking for a new place to plug it in." I plugged into my grandfather. He handed me principles that still shape my life:

1. Never leave a job, chore, or problem until it's settled or complete.
2. Every effort produces opportunity.
3. Mutual help, without expectation of pay, makes everyone stronger.

That foundation gave me the discipline to become a physician. It also made me a crusader, an adventurer, and a person who wouldn't let go of a question just because it was uncomfortable.

But no amount of grit prepared me for the slow death I witnessed in the medical profession.

At the peak of my private OB/GYN practice, I lost everything.

The financial collapse of my practice came swiftly and without warning. I had no idea what I had done wrong. There was no misconduct, no scandal, no violation of care. It happened because I didn't receive the one thing I never knew I needed: a business education. I blamed myself. Fully. The shame was immediate and crushing. With no income, no answers, and no clear path forward, I spiraled into suicidal thoughts. Divorce followed. The medical community I had loved turned its back. Friends disappeared. Even antidepressants couldn't dull the pain.

And yet, I couldn't let it go.

I knew I had done everything I was taught. But I began to wonder: What if the system had failed me, not the other way around?

That question led me to research. For the past 25 years, I've studied the one omission that has silently sabotaged physicians across the country: The complete absence of business education in medical school.

We are trained to practice medicine. We are not trained to sustain it.

No medical school in the United States or elsewhere in the world includes a formal curriculum in business education. Educators claim there isn't time. But we all know you can't master all of medicine in four years. So why have we accepted a model that leaves physicians uninformed about contracts, revenue cycles, debt management, and the fundamental skills required to run a practice?

This isn't just burnout. This is institutional design with no forethought.

Physicians around the globe experience the same consequences of a lack of business education. The lack of business education of the physician is called socialized medicine.

This book has detailed the steps that have taken American physicians from freedom to practice medicine as they choose to the socialized medicine system we see approaching us. A physician's loss of full control of their destiny in medicine destroys the profession.

If you don't understand business, you are vulnerable. Vulnerable to contracts that exploit you. To practice models that bleed you dry. To hospitals and health systems that view you as a number on a spreadsheet rather than a human being.

And what happens when physicians collapse under that weight? They leave. Or worse, they stay and grow numb. The loss is personal, but it is also systemic. The cost is not just to individual MDs but also to the very soul of medicine.

After losing my practice, I took a hospitalist job in another state. For five years, I endured the kind of conditions described throughout this book. Eventually, I left the field of medicine in 1999. It wasn't because I stopped loving my patients. It was because I could no longer endure a system that punished integrity and ignored reality.

I have been writing about the causes of and the solutions for our physician crisis for 25 years.

My goal is not to tear down medicine. My goal is to make it whole. To challenge the institutions that have normalized harm. To provide physicians with language to express what they are feeling. To show medical students that their humanity is not a liability. And to advocate for business education as a standard, not an exception.

I believe we are approaching a tipping point. With more physicians leaving practice, more medical students questioning the path, and more patients feeling the ripple effects, we can no longer pretend the system is sound.

This book was born from that urgency. It is my letter to those still inside medicine, and to those watching from the outside. It is a plea to listen. To rethink. To act.

I didn't write this epilogue to rehash my pain. I wrote it to say: I am still here. And so are you.

Others may have failed us. But we are not finished.

Let's build something better *together.*

—Dr. Graham

About the Author

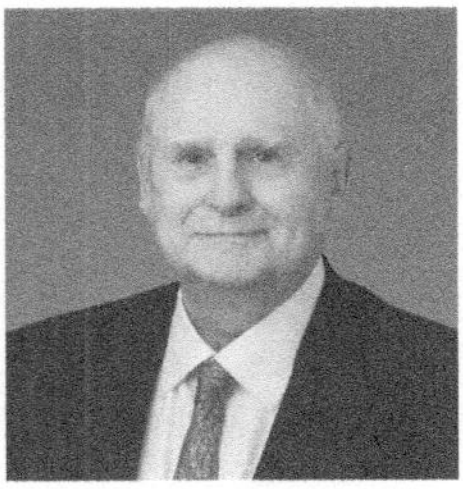

Curtis G. Graham, MD, ACOG, FACS is a rare combination of seasoned physician, medical practice expert, and medical business strategist. Over four decades in clinical practice, he pursued a demanding goal: to deliver the highest level of patient care while continually advancing his knowledge, skills, and methods. He embraced new surgical techniques, adopted emerging technologies, and encouraged physicians to educate patients more effectively about their conditions and treatments.

Dr. Graham's commitment to education began with patient handouts and expanded into articles, newsletters, and books addressing critical issues in modern healthcare. He has published more than 300 medical articles and several books focused on improving care delivery and physician sustainability. Alongside his clinical work, he studied practice management and communication with leading business educators, including Dan Kennedy, gaining insight into the nonclinical forces shaping modern medicine.

A turning point in his career came when he recognized the systemic roots of physician burnout and attrition: medical education does not adequately prepare physicians for the practical, financial, and administrative realities of modern practice. His work now focuses on addressing that gap.

Made in United States
Cleveland, OH
05 November 2026

47678347R00101